Primary Care

American Psychiatric Press
CONCISE GUIDES

Robert E. Hales, M.D.
Series Editor

CONCISE GUIDE TO

Psychiatry for Primary Care Practitioners

Michael F. Gliatto, M.D.
Stanley N. Caroff, M.D.
Robert Kaiser, M.D.

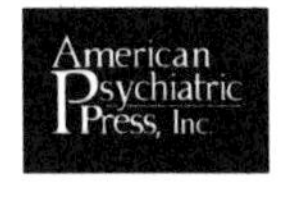

Washington, DC
London, England

Note: The authors have worked to ensure that all information in this book concerning drug dosages, schedules, and routes of administration is accurate as of the time of publication and consistent with standards set by the U.S. Food and Drug Administration and the general medical community. As medical research and practice advance, however, therapeutic standards may change. For this reason and because human and mechanical errors sometimes occur, we recommend that readers follow the advice of a physician who is directly involved in their care or the care of a member of their family.

Manufactured in the United States of America on acid-free paper
02 01 00 99 4 3 2 1

American Psychiatric Press, Inc.
1400 K Street, N.W.
Washington, DC 20005
www.appi.org

Library of Congress Cataloging-in-Publication Data
Concise guide to psychiatry for primary care practitioners / [edited by] Michael F. Gliatto, Stanley N. Caroff, Robert Kaiser.
p. cm. — (Concise guides / American Psychiatric Press)
Includes bibliographical references and index.
ISBN 0-88048-345-8
1. Psychiatry. 2. Primary care (Medicine). I. Gliatto, Michael F. II. Caroff, Stanley N., 1949- . III. Kaiser, Robert M. IV. Series: Concise guides (American Psychiatric Press)
[DNLM: 1. Mental Disorders—therapy. 2. Mental Disorders—diagnosis. 3. Psychotherapy—methods. 4. Primary Health Care—methods.
WM 140 C744 1999]
RC454.4.C66 1999
616.89—dc21
DNLM/DLC 98-32241
for Library of Congress CIP

British Library Cataloguing in Publication Data
A CIP record is available from the British Library.

CONTENTS

Contributors . . . . **xv**
Introduction to the American Psychiatric Press Concise Guides . . . . **xvii**
Preface . . . . **xix**

1 MOOD DISORDERS **1**
Howard J. Ilivicky, M.D.
TYPES OF DEPRESSION 2
Psychotic Depression 2
Melancholic Depression 3
Atypical Depression 3
Seasonal Depression 3
Postpartum Depression 4
Secondary Depression 4
Bipolar Disorder 4
Dysthymia. 6
Bereavement 6
COURSE OF ILLNESS AND PROGNOSIS. 7
EVALUATION 8
TREATMENT. 9
Medication. 10
Treatment Guidelines 18
Treatment Resistance 19
Nonpharmacological Treatment. 20
SPECIAL CLINICAL SITUATIONS 21
Geriatric Patients 21
Suicidal Patients. 22
CONCLUSION 22
REFERENCES. 22

2 ANXIETY DISORDERS 25
Nitin Kulkarni, M.D., and Richard J. Ross, M.D.
SPECIFIC ANXIETY DISORDERS 26
Panic Disorder 26
Phobias 29
Obsessive-Compulsive Disorder 31
Generalized Anxiety Disorder 31
Adjustment and Stress Disorders 32
Anxiety Disorder Due to a General Medical Condition 33
Substance-Induced Anxiety Disorders 34
COMORBIDITY 35
TREATMENT 36
Panic Disorder 37
Specific Phobia 41
Social Phobia 41
Obsessive-Compulsive Disorder 42
Generalized Anxiety Disorder 43
Stress Disorders 44
CONCLUSION 45
REFERENCES 45

3 SUBSTANCE USE DISORDERS 49
Wayne Barber, M.D.
GENERAL PRINCIPLES 49
GENERAL GUIDELINES FOR TREATMENT 52
SPECIFIC SUBSTANCES AND TREATMENT 53
Alcohol 53
Nicotine 65
Benzodiazepines 68
Substances Encountered Occasionally in Primary Care Settings 72
CONCLUSION 75
REFERENCES 75

4 **COGNITIVE DISORDERS. 77**
Michael F. Gliatto, M.D.
SPECIFIC DEMENTIAS 78
Alzheimer's Disease. 78
Vascular Dementia. 80
Subcortical Dementias 80
Dementia Secondary to Alcoholism 81
Other Irreversible Dementias 81
EVALUATION. 82
TREATMENT 86
Cognitive Symptoms 86
Associated Symptoms. 87
CONCLUSION 90
REFERENCES. 90

5 **SOMATOFORM AND RELATED DISORDERS. 93**
Sarah Gelbach DeMichele, M.D., and James L. Stinnett, M.D.
SPECIFIC SOMATOFORM DISORDERS 95
Somatization Disorder. 95
Conversion Disorder. 96
Hypochondriasis. 97
Body Dysmorphic Disorder 97
Pain Disorder 98
FACTITIOUS DISORDERS 98
MALINGERING 100
DELUSIONAL DISORDER 100
MANAGEMENT OF THE DOCTOR-PATIENT RELATIONSHIP IN PATIENTS WITH SOMATOFORM AND RELATED DISORDERS . . 100
CONCLUSION. 104
REFERENCES 104

6 **PSYCHOTIC DISORDERS** **107**
Stephan C. Mann, M.D., Michael F. Gliatto, M.D., E. Cabrina Campbell, M.D., and Robert A. Greenstein, M.D.
GENERAL CHARACTERISTICS 107
Delusions 107
Hallucinations 108
Disordered Thought Processes. 108
Disorganized Behavior. 109
Positive and Negative Symptoms 109
PSYCHOSIS ASSOCIATED WITH A MEDICAL CONDITION OR SUBSTANCE USE 109
General Medical Conditions 110
Substance-Induced Psychotic Disorders. 112
PSYCHOSIS ASSOCIATED WITH A PSYCHIATRIC DISORDER 112
Schizophrenia 116
Other Disorders 117
EVALUATION 119
ROLE OF PRIMARY CARE PRACTITIONERS 119
GENERAL PRINCIPLES OF TREATMENT 121
Antipsychotic Drugs 121
Treatment of Acute Psychosis 122
Maintenance Antipsychotic Drug Treatment 125
SIDE EFFECTS OF ANTIPSYCHOTICS. 126
Extrapyramidal Side Effects 126
Tardive Dyskinesia 127
Neuroleptic Malignant Syndrome 128
Other Side Effects 128
ATYPICAL AGENTS 130
CONCLUSION. 132
REFERENCES 132

7 DIFFICULT DOCTOR-PATIENT RELATIONSHIPS 135

Michael F. Gliatto, M.D.

PATIENT VARIABLES 135

Styles 135

Uncertain Diagnoses and Psychosocial Problems . . 138

EFFECT OF THESE VARIABLES ON THE DOCTOR-PATIENT RELATIONSHIP 140

SUGGESTIONS FOR TREATMENT 141

Initial Visit(s) 141

Later Visits 144

CONCLUSION 146

REFERENCES 146

8 SEXUAL DISORDERS 149

Mary F. Morrison, M.D., Antonio Fernando, M.D., and Monica Bishop, B.A.

HEALTHY SEXUAL FUNCTION 149

EVALUATION 150

Patient History 150

Medication History 152

Physical Examination 153

Laboratory Testing 153

SPECIFIC DISORDERS AND TREATMENT 155

Sexual Desire Disorders 155

Sexual Arousal Disorders 157

Orgasmic Disorders 160

Pain Disorders 162

Sexual Disorders in Selected Populations 164

CONCLUSION 165

REFERENCES 165

9 SLEEP DISORDERS. 169
Joyce R. Zinsenheim, M.D.
EVALUATION 170
SPECIFIC DISORDERS 170
Psychophysiological Insomnia. 170
Narcolepsy 171
Obstructive Sleep Apnea. 173
Periodic Limb Movements and Restless Legs Syndrome 175
Substance-Dependent Sleep Disorders 177
Circadian Rhythm Sleep Disorder. 178
Parasomnias 179
Sleep Disorders Associated With a Psychiatric Disorder 180
Sleep Disorders Associated With a Medical Disorder 180
TREATMENT 181
Use of Sedative-Hypnotics. 181
Other Treatments. 183
CONCLUSION. 183
REFERENCES 185

10 EATING AND WEIGHT DISORDERS 187
Barbara J. Wingate, M.D., John P. O'Reardon, M.D., and Thomas A. Wadden, Ph.D.
EATING DISORDERS. 187
Anorexia Nervosa 188
Bulimia Nervosa 191
TREATMENT OF EATING DISORDERS 193
General Principles 193
Anorexia Nervosa 194
Bulimia Nervosa 195
WEIGHT DISORDERS 196
TREATMENT OF WEIGHT DISORDERS 197
CONCLUSION. 197
REFERENCES 198

11 SUICIDE AND VIOLENCE. 199
E. Cabrina Campbell, M.D., Stephan C. Mann, M.D., Michael F. Gliatto, M.D., and Sheryl D. Hunter, M.D.
SUICIDE 199
Psychiatric Disorders 201
Medical Disorders 201
Evaluation 202
Treatment. 203
Medications 205
VIOLENCE. 205
Violence in Patients With Psychiatric Disorders . . 206
Evaluation 207
Domestic Violence 209
Treatment. 209
CONCLUSION. 210
REFERENCES 210

INDEX 213

LIST OF TABLES AND FIGURE

TABLES

Table 1–1 DSM-IV criteria for major depression 2
Table 1–2 Medical conditions associated with major depression 5
Table 1–3 Medications that may precipitate major depression 6
Table 1–4 DSM-IV criteria for manic episode 7
Table 1–5 Risk factors associated with depression 9
Table 1–6 Dosages of commonly prescribed antidepressants 12
Table 2–1 Characteristic symptoms of the anxiety disorders. 27
Table 2–2 Medications used to treat anxiety disorders . . . 38
Table 2–3 Benzodiazepines commonly used to treat anxiety disorders 40
Table 3–1 DSM-IV criteria for substance dependence . . . 50
Table 3–2 DSM-IV criteria for substance abuse. 51
Table 3–3 Signs and symptoms of intoxication 54
Table 3–4 Signs and symptoms of withdrawal 56
Table 3–5 Abnormal findings in heavy users of alcohol . . 59
Table 3–6 Interactions between alcohol and common medications 60
Table 3–7 Medications used to treat substance abuse 62
Table 3–8 Resources for smoking cessation 66
Table 4–1 Common causes of dementia 79
Table 4–2 Laboratory tests for the evaluation of dementia. 85
Table 4–3 Medications used to treat symptoms associated with dementia 88
Table 5–1 Somatoform and related disorders 94
Table 5–2 Treatment recommendations for patients with somatoform and related disorders 102

Table 6–1 Selected causes of psychotic disorder due to a general medical condition 111
Table 6–2 Selected causes of substance-induced psychotic disorder 113
Table 6–3 Abbreviated DSM-IV criteria for schizophrenia 117
Table 6–4 Antipsychotic drugs currently available in the United States 123
Table 7–1 Treatment recommendations for different patient styles 139
Table 7–2 Suggestions for working with patients 142
Table 8–1 Screening tool for sexual dysfunction. 152
Table 8–2 Physical examination to assess for sexual dysfunction. 154
Table 8–3 Recommended laboratory tests for evaluation of sexual dysfunction 155
Table 9–1 Sleep inventory 171
Table 9–2 Clinical features of the sleep disorders and their treatment 172
Table 9–3 Sleep hygiene recommendations 182
Table 9–4 Guidelines for the use of hypnotics 182
Table 9–5 Commonly used hypnotics 182
Table 9–6 Hypnotics with troublesome side effects 184
Table 10–1 DSM-IV criteria for anorexia nervosa 189
Table 10–2 Topics to consider when evaluating patients with eating and weight disorders 190
Table 10–3 Laboratory tests recommended for patients with eating disorders. 191
Table 10–4 DSM-IV criteria for bulimia nervosa 192
Table 11–1 Risk factors for suicide 200
Table 11–2 Psychiatric disorders associated with an increased risk for suicide. 201
Table 11–3 The SAD PERSONS Scale 203

Table 11–4 Scoring and treatment planning using the SAD PERSONS Scale 204
Table 11–5 Short-term risk factors for suicide. 205
Table 11–6 Risk factors for violent behavior 207
Table 11–7 Neuropsychiatric disorders associated with aggression 208
Table 11–8 Situations requiring a screen for physical abuse 209
Table 11–9 Medications used to treat aggression 210

FIGURE

Figure 4–1 Mini-Mental State Exam 84

CONTRIBUTORS

Wayne Barber, M.D.
Medical Director, Rehoboth McKinley Christian Health Care Services, Gallup, New Mexico

Monica Bishop, B.A.
Research Assistant, Department of Psychiatry, University of Pennsylvania School of Medicine, Philadelphia, Pennsylvania

E. Cabrina Campbell, M.D.
Assistant Professor of Psychiatry, University of Pennsylvania School of Medicine, Philadelphia, Pennsylvania

Stanley N. Caroff, M.D.
Professor of Psychiatry, University of Pennsylvania School of Medicine, Philadelphia, Pennsylvania

Sarah Gelbach DeMichele, M.D.
Assistant Professor of Psychiatry, University of Pennsylvania School of Medicine, Philadelphia, Pennsylvania

Antonio Fernando, M.D.
Assistant Instructor of Psychiatry, University of Pennsylvania School of Medicine, Philadelphia, Pennsylvania

Michael F. Gliatto, M.D.
Clinical Assistant Professor of Psychiatry, University of Pennsylvania School of Medicine, Philadelphia, Pennsylvania

Robert A. Greenstein, M.D.
Associate Professor in Psychiatry, University of Pennsylvania School of Medicine, Philadelphia, Pennsylvania

Sheryl D. Hunter, M.D.
Assistant Instructor of Psychiatry, University of Pennsylvania School of Medicine, Philadelphia, Pennsylvania

Howard J. Ilivicky, M.D.
Assistant Professor of Psychiatry, University of Pennsylvania School of Medicine, Philadelphia, Pennsylvania

Robert Kaiser, M.D.
Assistant Professor of Medicine, University of Pennsylvania School of Medicine, Philadelphia, Pennsylvania

Nitin Kulkarni, M.D.
Assistant Instructor of Psychiatry, University of Pennsylvania School of Medicine, Philadelphia, Pennsylvania

Stephan C. Mann, M.D.
Associate Professor of Psychiatry, University of Pennsylvania School of Medicine, Philadelphia, Pennsylvania

Mary F. Morrison, M.D.
Assistant Professor of Psychiatry, University of Pennsylvania School of Medicine, Philadelphia, Pennsylvania

John P. O'Reardon, M.D.
Assistant Instructor of Psychiatry, University of Pennsylvania School of Medicine, Philadelphia, Pennsylvania

Richard J. Ross, M.D.
Associate Professor of Psychiatry, University of Pennsylvania School of Medicine, Philadelphia, Pennsylvania

James L. Stinnett, M.D.
Professor of Psychiatry, University of Pennsylvania School of Medicine, Philadelphia, Pennsylvania

Thomas A. Wadden, Ph.D.
Professor of Psychology in Psychiatry, University of Pennsylvania School of Medicine, Philadelphia, Pennsylvania

Barbara J. Wingate, M.D.
Assistant Professor of Psychiatry, University of Pennsylvania School of Medicine, Philadelphia, Pennsylvania

Joyce R. Zinsenheim, M.D.
Instructor of Psychiatry, University of Pennsylvania School of Medicine, Philadelphia, Pennsylvania

INTRODUCTION

to the American Psychiatric Press Concise Guides

The American Psychiatric Press *Concise Guides* series provides practical information for psychiatrists, psychiatry residents, and medical students working in a variety of treatment settings, such as inpatient psychiatry units, outpatient clinics, consultation-liaison services, or private office settings. The *Concise Guides* are meant to complement the more detailed information to be found in lengthier psychiatry texts.

The *Concise Guides* address topics of special concern to psychiatrists in clinical practice. The books in this series contain a detailed table of contents, along with an index, tables, figures, and other charts for easy access. The books are designed to fit into a lab coat pocket or jacket pocket, which makes them a convenient source of information. References have been limited to those most relevant to the material presented.

This *Concise Guide to Psychiatry for Primary Care Practitioners* is a practical, user-friendly guide for primary care physicians to use when dealing with psychiatric disorders or behavioral problems in their ambulatory care patients. The editors and all of the authors except one are faculty members at the University of Pennsylvania either in the Department of Psychiatry or the Department of Internal Medicine. The editors have prepared a first-rate guide that includes the most common psychiatric disorders encountered in primary care practice: mood disorders, anxiety disorders, and substance use disorders. It also includes other disorders that are frequently treated by primary care physicians: cognitive disorders, somatoform disorders, psychotic disorders, sexual disorders, sleep disorders, and eating disorders. The chapters that focus on psychiatric disorders include a number of helpful tables that summarize diagnostic, assessment, and treatment issues. All of the chapters include relevant references that the reader may turn to for more detailed information.

In addition, the guide includes two very helpful chapters that primary care physicians should find particularly useful. Chapter 7, "Difficult Doctor-Patient Relationships," by Dr. Michael F. Gliatto, is an especially compelling chapter that uses case vignettes to illustrate important teaching points. Dr. Gliatto also provides very helpful suggestions for physicians to consider when faced with patients who may be difficult to manage. The final chapter, on suicide and violence, by Drs. Campbell, Mann, and Hunter, is an equally helpful chapter that provides guidance of relevance to primary care physicians in anticipating and preventing both suicide and violence.

In summary, Drs. Gliatto, Caroff, and Kaiser have edited an outstanding guide to which primary care physicians may refer when managing psychiatric disorders in their patients. Given that the majority of psychiatric care today is provided in ambulatory, primary care settings, it is appropriate that an outstanding guide has been prepared to assist primary care physicians with the challenging task of managing such patients.

Robert E. Hales, M.D., M.B.A.
Series Editor
American Psychiatric Press
Concise Guides

PREFACE

By necessity and tradition, primary care practitioners have always been asked to help patients and families deal with primary emotional problems or reactions to medical illnesses. Because of denial and a fear of social stigmatization, many patients with mental illnesses are more likely to seek treatment from their family doctor. As a result of continuing changes in the provision and reimbursement of medical and psychiatric care, primary care practitioners may be expected to manage, or at least competently screen, even more patients who have complex and serious mental disorders before referring them to a psychiatrist.

Many practitioners may be uncomfortable managing psychiatric disorders. They may not be up to date on recent advances in psychiatry. Symptoms of many primarily behavioral disorders may be subtle, and the medical and pharmacological etiology of other syndromes can be easily overlooked—to the detriment of the patient. Psychopharmacology has become more complex as a result of the proliferation of the drugs available, their widespread use, and their potential toxicity. The theory and practice of the psychotherapies are obscure to most practitioners in primary care, and these highly effective modalities remain beyond the expertise and the time available to most clinicians.

The discrepancy between clinicians' skills and patients' needs—which may have serious consequences for the effectiveness, efficiency, and safety of mental health care—prompted us to write this guide. It is designed as a quick reference to help primary care practitioners better understand, diagnose, and initially manage the mental illnesses they are likely to encounter in an office practice. This guide is the result of a collaborative effort by experienced psychiatrists who have a range of general and specialized interests in psychiatry and medicine. It provides a brief, readable, jargon-free, and pragmatic overview of selected, common conditions to enable practitioners to elicit a relevant history, perform a competent mental status examination, and recognize signs of psychiatric illnesses. Management techniques appropriate for outpatient practice are suggested, with an emphasis on when to seek consultation with psychiatric colleagues.

This guide is not meant to be comprehensive. References are listed to allow for further study. Disorders that occur mainly in hospitalized patients or that present in emergency settings are discussed only briefly. Although disorders of personality represent a significant cause of psychiatric morbidity, we have focused only on how these disorders appear within, and potentially threaten, the doctor- patient relationship.

Dramatic progress has been made over the past few decades, and the chances for the mentally ill to have a normal life in the community have improved dramatically. The guiding principle of this guide was the preservation of these advances by fostering an active collaboration between primary care practitioners and psychiatrists.

We wish to acknowledge the assistance of Charlene Johnson and Joanne Loguidice in preparing the manuscript for publication. We dedicate the book to our families for their support, and to our patients from whom we have much more to learn.

Michael F. Gliatto, M.D.
Stanley N. Caroff, M.D.
Robert Kaiser, M.D.

1

MOOD DISORDERS

Howard J. Ilivicky, M.D.

Clinical depression is a common illness often seen in the primary care setting. Approximately 60% of patients with major depression will seek professional help from primary care practitioners rather than mental health professionals (1). With proper diagnosis of the depression, appropriate use of antidepressant medication, and short-term supportive psychotherapy, many patients in the ambulatory setting can be treated successfully and have improved mental, physical, and social functioning (2).

Mood disorders remain poorly recognized as syndromal illnesses characterized by a constellation of signs and symptoms. Depression has no biological markers on which to base the diagnosis. The practitioner must rely on the medical interview and make the diagnosis using DSM-IV (3) criteria, which can be remembered by applying the mnemonic SIG: E CAPS (i.e., prescribe energy capsules) (see Table 1–1) (4).

Major depression occurs in 2%–4% of the general population, in 5%–10% of outpatient primary care patients, and in 10%–14% of medical inpatients (5). In each setting, even more people will have a depressed mood or any of the symptoms listed in Table 1–1 but not meet the DSM-IV criteria for major depression.

The societal burden of depression is great. The estimated cost of mood disorders in the United States is $43 billion per year (6). Depressed patients have more medical illnesses than those without the disorder, and they use health care services at higher rates (6). The identification and treatment of depression will thus reduce medical care costs.

TABLE 1–1. **DSM-IV criteria for major depression**	
Sleep	Insomnia
Interests	Loss of interest or pleasure in activities
Guilt	Excessive guilt, worthlessness, hopelessness
Energy	Loss of energy or fatigue
Concentration	Diminished concentration ability, indecisiveness
Appetite	Decreased appetite, 5% weight loss or gain
Psychomotor	Psychomotor retardation or agitation
Suicidality	Suicidal thoughts, ideation, plan, or attempt; includes thoughts of death or preoccupation with death

Source. Reprinted from Wise MG, Rundell JR: *Concise Guide to Consultation Psychiatry,* 2nd Edition. Washington, DC, American Psychiatric Press, 1994, p. 56. Used with permission.

In this chapter, I review diagnostic considerations, treatment options, and the role of psychiatric consultation in managing mood disorders. The practitioner then will be able to recognize various mood disorders and improve patient care.

■ TYPES OF DEPRESSION

Studies of major depression reveal heterogeneity with regard to biology, family history, pharmacological response, genetics, and course of illness. Several schemes have been proposed to subdivide major depression. Although the subgroups may not be all-inclusive or etiologically distinct, they often have implications for treatment selection and prognosis.

Psychotic Depression

The term *psychotic features* refers to the presence of delusions or hallucinations. In psychotic depressions, psychotic features are never present without concurrent mood symptoms. The depressive symptoms are severe and occur before the onset of psychosis. Usually, the contents of the delusions or hallucinations (called *mood-congruent psychotic symptoms*) are consistent with the predominant mood. For example, a patient may have a delusion that he or she has sinned in an unforgivable way. Treatment requires an antidepressant medication plus an antipsychotic (7).

Melancholic Depression

Melancholia is a severe form of depression seen more commonly in older patients. The essential features include psychomotor retardation or agitation, loss of interest or pleasure, lack of reactivity to usually pleasant stimuli, depression that is worse in the morning than in the evening (*diurnal variation*), and early morning awakening. These symptoms appear to repeat from episode to episode and may be misdiagnosed as dementia. Antidepressant medication is mandatory treatment. If medications fail, electroconvulsive therapy (ECT) should be strongly considered for these patients (7).

Atypical Depression

Atypical features are named for their apparent contradiction to the criteria list for major depression. Features include overeating/weight gain, oversleeping, a mood that still responds to events (*reactive mood*), extreme sensitivity to interpersonal rejection, and a feeling of heaviness in the arms and legs (*leaden paralysis*). These symptoms are more common in younger patients. Medication trials suggest the effectiveness of certain classes of antidepressants, for example, selective serotonin reuptake inhibitors (SSRIs) and monoamine oxidase inhibitors (MAOIs).

Seasonal Depression

Seasonal depression involves recurrent episodes of depression that have a regular temporal relationship between the onset of the episode and a particular period of the year (such as onset in the fall and remission in the spring). Light therapy, in which patients are exposed to a standard fluorescent lighting apparatus, may be effective for treating mild to moderate disorders.

Postpartum Depression

Postpartum mood symptoms are divided into three categories: blues, psychosis, and depression. Postpartum blues are brief episodes (lasting 1–4 days) of fluctuating mood and tearfulness that frequently occur within several days after delivery. Treatment consists of reassurance and time.

The incidence of postpartum psychosis is low. The symptoms typically begin 2–3 days after delivery. Features can include disorientation, extreme agitation, emotional lability, and psychotic symptoms. Although the prognosis is generally good, a rare complication is infanticide or suicide. Postpartum depressions meeting severity levels for major depression have a prevalence of 10%–15% within the first 3–6 months after childbirth as compared with expected rates of 5%–7% in nonchildbearing matched control subjects (7). Patients with a psychiatric history are particularly at risk. There is a 50% chance of recurrence of postpartum psychosis in the next postpartum period (7). Episodes of postpartum psychosis and postpartum depression require medication and often hospitalization.

Secondary Depression

Between 5% and 10% of patients who meet criteria for major depression actually have a mood syndrome caused by underlying medical disease (see Table 1–2), medications (see Table 1–3), or substance abuse (1). Each of these conditions would then be called mood disorder due to a general medical condition or substance-induced mood disorder. A thorough medical history, a physical examination, a review of medications, and appropriate laboratory tests help to rule out causes of secondary depression. Depressive symptoms may occur in up to 30% of persons who abuse alcohol (8).

Bipolar Disorder

Bipolar disorder features episodes of major depression interspersed with episodes of mania and/or hypomania. Manic episodes

TABLE 1–2. **Medical conditions associated with major depression**

Central nervous system

Alzheimer's disease, AIDS dementia complex, brain tumors, multiple sclerosis, Huntington's disease, stroke, head injury, Parkinson's disease

Endocrine

Hypothyroidism, Cushing's syndrome, diabetes mellitus, Addison's disease, apathetic hyperthyroidism

Autoimmune

Rheumatoid arthritis, systemic lupus erythematosus

Other

Pancreatic cancer, chronic pain syndrome, fibromyalgia, chronic fatigue syndrome

Note. AIDS = acquired immunodeficiency syndrome.
Source. Adapted from Salazar 1996 (1).

are distinct periods, lasting at least 1 week (with hypomania for at least 4 days), of persistently elevated, abnormally expansive, or irritable mood. Associated features can include inflated self-esteem, rapid speech, racing internal thoughts, marked distractibility, decreased need for sleep, increased goal-directed activity, and involvement in pleasurable activities without regard for negative consequences (e.g., buying sprees or sexual indiscretions) (3). The mnemonic GIDDINESS, as delineated in Table 1–4 (4), can be used to remember these criteria.

Mixed episodes commonly occur, wherein the patient simultaneously experiences the symptoms of mania and depression. The lifetime prevalence of bipolar disorder in community samples is 0.4%–1.6% (3). The significance of identifying patients who have bipolar disorder is that treatment with an antidepressant for a major depressive episode can precipitate or worsen manic symptoms.

Standard treatment involves first starting a patient on a mood-stabilizing agent. The three standard agents are lithium carbonate, valproic acid, and carbamazepine. If a patient with a history of bipolar disorder is in the depressed phase, an antidepressant will

TABLE 1–3. **Medications that may precipitate major depression**

Anti-inflammatory agents	
	Indomethacin, phenacetin, phenylbutazone, pentazocine
Antihypertensive agents	
	Clonidine, methyldopa, reserpine, hydralazine, propranolol, prazosin
Cardiovascular agents	
	Digitalis, procainamide
Central nervous system agents	
	Amantadine, L-dopa, barbiturates, carbamazepine
Hormones	
	Corticosteroids, estrogen, progesterone, birth control pills

Source. Adapted from Salazar 1996 (1).

need to be started in addition to the mood stabilizer. If the mania is severe, psychotic symptoms may develop; neuroleptics are then indicated. Benzodiazepines are useful to help treat the agitation that may be present along with the mania. Patients with bipolar disorder should be referred to a psychiatrist.

Dysthymia

Dysthymic disorder, also called *dysthymia,* is a chronic sadness lasting at least 2 consecutive years and associated with at least two of the symptoms of a major depressive episode although not meeting full criteria for a major depressive episode. Most individuals with dysthymia go on to develop major depression. Dysthymia appears to respond to a variety of antidepressant agents, which can reduce dramatically the morbidity associated with this insidious disorder (9).

Bereavement

Bereavement is a natural human reaction to the death of a loved one. The bereaved individual often can exhibit all the symptoms of a major depressive episode. The individual typically regards the

TABLE 1–4. **DSM-IV criteria for manic episode**

Grandiosity
Increased activity
Decreased judgment (risky activities)
Distractibility
Irritability
Need for sleep decreased
Elevated mood
Speedy thoughts
Speedy talk

Source. Reprinted from Wise MG, Rundell JR: *Concise Guide to Consultation Psychiatry,* 2nd Edition. Washington, DC, American Psychiatric Press, 1994, p. 67. Used with permission.

depressed mood as normal. The diagnosis of major depression is not given unless the symptoms are still present 2 months after the loss or if certain symptoms not characteristic of a normal grief reaction are present. These symptoms include the following: 1) exaggerated guilt, 2) thoughts of death other than the survivor's feeling that he or she should have died with or instead of the deceased person, 3) preoccupation with worthlessness, 4) marked psychomotor retardation, 5) severe functional impairment, and 6) hallucinatory experiences other than transiently hearing the voice of, or seeing the image of, the deceased person (3). Professional help may be sought for the relief of symptoms such as insomnia, decreased appetite, or weight loss but should definitely be sought when a depressive episode is in full course.

■ COURSE OF ILLNESS AND PROGNOSIS

For most people, major depression is a lifelong, episodic disorder with multiple recoveries and recurrences, averaging one episode per 5-year period (10). Most episodes of depression resolve within 6–8 months, although 10% of depressed individuals will not recover from an episode. Because of recurrences and lack of recovery, approximately 20% of patients with major depression experience a chronic, unremitting course. The long-term functional effects of major depression and depressive symptoms persist even beyond the resolution of acute symptoms. Individuals are likely to have ongoing limitations in physical activities, employment difficulties, poor spousal relationships, less satisfactory sexual activity, and increased risk of suicide.

Clinical variables can be predictive of illness course. An increased number of prior episodes and the presence of secondary depression predict increased relapse rates (10). Half of persons who have one depressive episode are likely to have at least one recurrence in their lifetime. The risk of recurrence increases thereafter: 70% after two depressive episodes and 90% after three episodes (11). The most reliable predictors of symptom persistence are duration of symptoms of prior episodes, depression associated with a medical illness (10), and symptom severity. Demographic variables are not consistent predictors of illness course. Treatment can profoundly alter these outcomes. Multiple goals of treatment include shortening recovery time (usually to within 4–8 weeks), decreasing recurrences, improving function, and decreasing morbidity and mortality.

■ EVALUATION

Primary care practitioners fail to make a diagnosis in as many as 50%–70% of the patients who present to them with mood disorders (12, 13). Individuals whose depression is not diagnosed tend to have milder symptoms, but depression also is missed in those with severe symptoms. Many symptoms of depression are similar to those seen in medical illnesses. The practitioner should have a high index of suspicion when patients report poorly defined or multiple somatic symptoms such as chronic pain (especially headaches) unresponsive to appropriate analgesics, anxiety, fatigue, sleep disturbances, sexual complaints, tinnitus, or bouts of diarrhea alternating with those of constipation (1). Familiarity with the risk factors associated with depression (see Table 1–5) may help practitioners to

TABLE 1–5. **Risk factors associated with depression**

Gender (females are more likely than males to be depressed)
Age (peak occurrence: female, age 35–45 years; male, age >55 years)
Stressful life events
Lack of social support (especially if unmarried)
History of depression
Family history of depression or suicide
Medical comorbidity
Lower socioeconomic status
Concurrent substance abuse
Postpartum period
Comorbid anxiety

identify patients who have depression (1).Warranting particular attention is the occurrence of anxiety in the ambulatory setting. Half of depressed patients exhibit symptoms of anxiety (1). Misdiagnosing depression as anxiety is a common error, even for psychiatrists.

In suspected cases of major depression, the diagnosis of depression should not be excluded simply because the patient denies feeling depressed (1). The elderly, men, and African Americans are less likely to acknowledge depressive symptoms or receive care for depression (14). Socioeconomic variables have not been consistently reported to be factors in patients' reporting of mood symptoms (14). Other obstacles to the appropriate recognition of depression by practitioners are inadequate knowledge of diagnostic criteria, competing comorbid conditions, time limitations in busy office settings, concerns about the implications of labeling, and poor reimbursement mechanisms (15).

■ TREATMENT

Depression can be treated successfully in primary care clinics as long as clinicians understand the situations requiring psychiatric intervention. Primary care practitioners should treat patients who have depressive symptoms but who do not have severe functional impairment or suicidal ideation. They should try one course of an SSRI at the maximum dosage, if necessary. If the symptoms remain refractory or worsen, psychiatric referral is warranted. A psychiatrist should be consulted for the use of MAOIs, tricyclic antidepressants (TCAs), or augmenting strategies. I discuss these approaches later in this chapter.

Consultation should also be used to verify the diagnosis, to consider other mental and medical disorders that may be in the differential diagnosis, and to give specific recommendations for psychopharmacological and psychotherapeutic interventions. Complex psychosocial factors can interfere with treatment and often require a psychiatric team approach for successful intervention. Psychiatric referral should also be sought if the patient requests it.

Patients with severe forms of depression require psychiatric hospitalization. These forms include conditions in which active suicidality, severe psychosis, or extreme decreases in level of functioning are present. Patients with bipolar disorder also benefit from hospitalization when they are unstable.

Medication

Antidepressant medication is the first line of pharmacotherapy for patients with major depression, especially if their symptoms are moderate to severe, incapacitating, chronic, or recurrent; if they have a family history of depression; or if they have a personal or family history of responding to antidepressants. The presence of psychotic, melancholic, or atypical symptoms also indicates a need for medication. When patients do not have all of the symptoms of major depression, it is less obvious that medications are superior to treatment with placebo combined with minimally supportive measures (16). When mood symptoms are mild, it is best to wait before prescribing an antidepressant; some of these patients will go on to develop major depression, at which point they will require treatment (9, 14).

Population studies show that all antidepressants are equally effective, but response may vary from one patient to another (1, 16). Significant symptom improvement occurs in 40%–80% of patients taking medication (7). Inadequate drug dosage or treatment duration is the most common reason for suboptimal or partial response to antidepressant treatment. Only 20%–40% of patients who were prescribed antidepressants (usually TCAs) received dosages above established minimums (17, 18). Approximately one-third of depressed primary care patients discontinue antidepressant medication within the first month of treatment (1, 18). The reasons patients give for stopping medications include unpleasant side effects, worsening of depressive symptoms, and early recovery (17). Table 1–6 provides some guidelines for the medications discussed in the following sections (19, 20).

Selective serotonin reuptake inhibitors. The SSRIs and the TCAs are equally efficacious (21). The SSRIs are a good choice for treating an episode of depression because of favorable side-effect profiles, effectiveness in treating all types of depression, and tolerability with comorbid medical conditions. These medications increase serotonin in the central nervous system. Three commonly prescribed SSRIs are fluoxetine (Prozac), sertraline (Zoloft), and paroxetine (Paxil). With the exception of sertraline, therapy can be initiated at therapeutic dosages: fluoxetine at 20 mg/day and paroxetine at 20 mg/day. The recommended starting dosage for sertraline is 50 mg/day, but at least 100 mg/day is usually needed to achieve a response. The dosage can usually be increased at the beginning of the second week of therapy. Blood level monitoring is also unnecessary. These medications have the advantage of once-daily dosing. Fluoxetine should be given only in the morning (because it may cause insomnia), whereas sertraline and paroxetine can be given at night depending on the patient's reaction. If sleep disruption occurs, the medication should be given in the morning.

Atypical depression is particularly responsive to the SSRIs. Delusional depression requires the combination of an SSRI and an

TABLE 1–6. **Dosages of commonly prescribed antidepressants**

Medication	Initial dosage	Incremental change[a]	Usual therapeutic dosage (mg/day)	Maximum recommended dosage (mg/day)
Fluoxetine (Prozac)	10–20 mg/day[b]	20 mg/day for 3 weeks; then increase by 20 mg/day every 3–4 weeks	20–60	80
Paroxetine (Paxil)	20 mg/day[c]	20 mg/day for 2–3 weeks; then increase by 10–20 mg/day each week	20–50	50
Sertraline (Zoloft)	50 mg/day[d]	50 mg/day for 3–4 weeks; then increase by 50 mg/day each week until 200-mg/day dosage is reached	50–200	200
Fluvoxamine (Luvox)	50–100 mg/day	Increase by 50 mg/day every 4–7 days[e]	100–200	300
Nefazodone (Serzone)	50 mg bid	Increase by 50 mg/day every 4 days to 200 mg/day; then increase by 100–400 mg/day each week; maintain this dosage for 3–4 weeks[f]	300–500	600
Venlafaxine (Effexor)	18.75 mg bid[g]	Increase by 18.75 mg every 3 days to 32.5 mg bid; then increase by 37.5 mg every 3 days or 75 mg/week until 150-mg/day dosage is reached[h]	75–225	375
Bupropion (Wellbutrin)	100 mg bid	Increase to 100 mg tid by day 4[i]	300–400	450

Mirtazepine (Remeron)	7.5 mg/day	Increase to 15 mg/day after 3–4 days	15–45	45

Note. [a]These increments are to be based on clinical response. If a patient responds at an initial dosage, then the patient should remain at that dosage for the duration of the trial or until the dosage proves to be ineffective. [b]A suspension is available so that dosages as low as 2 mg/day can be given. Geriatric patients should start at 5–10 mg/day. [c]Tablets are scored. Geriatric patients should start at 10 mg/day. [d]It is cheaper to prescribe the scored 100-mg tablets; the tablets can be broken in half for 50-mg dosages. Start geriatric patients at 25 mg/day. [e]For dosages greater than 100 mg/day, use a bid schedule. [f]If there is no response after week 4, increase the daily dosage by 100 mg/day each week until a dosage of 500–600 mg/day is reached. [g]Geriatric patients should start at 12.5 mg/day. [h]Beyond 150 mg/day, increase dosage 75 mg/day each week until 225 mg/day is reached. If ineffective, the dosage should be tapered over 2–3 weeks. [i]Single doses should not exceed 150 mg.

antipsychotic medication. Patients with mood symptoms that do not meet the criteria for major depression but who have significant functional impairment will also respond to the SSRIs. The SSRIs also are used to treat psychiatric disorders that frequently coexist with depression, including obsessive-compulsive disorder, post-traumatic stress disorder, panic disorder, and eating disorders.

The SSRIs are particularly useful in treating depression in the elderly and in patients who have concurrent medical illness. They do not cause autonomic or cardiovascular adverse effects. The SSRIs are the agents of choice for depressed patients who have heart conduction disease, orthostatic hypotension, ventricular arrhythmias, or ischemic heart disease. Sinus-node slowing is the only reported cardiovascular side effect (9). The relative lack of adverse effects accounts for the wide therapeutic index of the SSRIs and makes them relatively safe in overdosage situations.

The SSRIs do have side effects that result from overstimulation of the serotonin system. These effects include insomnia, agitation, nervousness, headaches, gastrointestinal disturbances (especially nausea), and sexual dysfunction. Most of these disturbances are transient and resolve within the first few weeks of treatment, although sexual side effects may persist. Insomnia can be treated with sedatives. Drug holidays during an SSRI regimen may be useful.

All SSRIs inhibit hepatic microsomal cytochrome P450 drug-metabolizing enzymes. Patients who are receiving concomitant therapy with drugs metabolized by the cytochrome P450 enzyme system should be monitored for potential drug interactions with the SSRIs. Although there has been some concern that the SSRIs interact with the antihistamine astemizole (Hismanal) to produce cardiotoxicity, it is now felt that clinically significant antihistamine accumulation does not occur with therapeutic dosages of the SSRIs. However, the manufacturer of Zoloft (sertraline) recently changed the package insert to warn of this potential interaction (22). There have also been reports of increased plasma concentrations of TCAs and alprazolam (Xanax) following cytochrome P450 inhibition by the SSRIs.

Differences in the pharmacokinetic properties of the SSRIs also can have important clinical implications. Fluoxetine and its metabolite norfluoxetine have long half-lives and may take up to 80 days to be eliminated completely from the body. This property may become important if a change in drug therapy is required. Sertraline has a minimally active metabolite, whereas paroxetine does not have an active metabolite. Therefore, one must wait 2 weeks between stopping sertraline or paroxetine and starting an MAOI, whereas one must wait 6 weeks after fluoxetine is stopped (1, 2).

Appropriate concern exists over the cost of the newer antidepressant agents, including the SSRIs; however, the overall cost of treatment may be reduced when a full course of a more expensive medication with a narrower side-effect profile leads to a higher rate of success. Patients treated with the newer antidepressants are significantly more likely to continue treatment past 30 days, to fill four or more prescriptions within a 6-month follow-up period, and to reach an adequate daily dosage (17, 18).

Bupropion. Bupropion (Wellbutrin) is an antidepressant with different neurochemical properties than those of other available antidepressant drugs. Its putative mechanism of action involves dopamine and norepinephrine reuptake inhibition. Bupropion is an effective alternative for patients who are unable to tolerate the SSRIs. It is not associated with sexual dysfunction, and it has a low incidence of cardiovascular side effects, orthostatic hypotension, and anticholinergic effects. Bupropion may be added to a trial of an SSRI to treat sexual dysfunction associated with the SSRIs (23). With its mild stimulatory effects, it is also a particularly useful agent in lethargic, depressed elderly patients.

Anecdotal evidence indicates that bupropion is useful for patients who have bipolar disorder, because the medication is associated with a lower incidence of secondary mania (9). The primary concern with this medication is its potential for inducing seizures, which increases with dosages greater than 450 mg/day or when one single dose is greater than 150 mg. Bupropion should not be given to patients who have a known seizure disorder or a potential seizure focus. Other side effects include nausea, insomnia, anxiety, agitation, and hypertension. Because of its short half-life, bupropion is given two to three times a day with a dosage range of 300–450 mg/day.

Nefazodone. Nefazodone (Serzone) is a recently approved antidepressant that is a potent antagonist of serotonin postsynaptic receptors and an inhibitor of the reuptake of serotonin and norepinephrine. Its efficacy is comparable to that of other antidepressants. Although nefazodone has some of the side effects of the SSRIs and the TCAs, the effects are much less severe with nefazodone. In particular, nefazodone has a low incidence of sexual dysfunction. It has a short half-life and requires twice-a-day dosing with a usual effective dosage range of 300–600 mg/day. Nefazodone use is contraindicated with terfenadine (Seldane), which has been withdrawn from the market, and with astemizole because of cardiotoxic effects; and it has potential interactions with alprazolam and triazolam (Halcion) (22).

Venlafaxine. Venlafaxine (Effexor), another relatively new agent, selectively inhibits norepinephrine, serotonin, and dopamine. Because of the cardiovascular side effects and significant nausea associated with its use, it is not considered a first-line agent. Hypertension is especially common when dosages of 375 mg/day or more are used. Patients should have regular blood pressure checks when taking venlafaxine, particularly when dosages are changed. Therapeutic dosages usually are 75–225 mg/day, and the medication requires twice- or thrice-daily dosing, which further limits its usefulness.

Mirtazepine. Mirtazepine (Remeron), the most recent antidepressant to be marketed in the United States, is a direct antagonist of serotonin and norepinephrine α_2 receptors. Mirtazepine represents another reasonable alternative for the depressed patient who is not responsive to the SSRIs (24).

Tricyclic antidepressants. The TCAs influence the reuptake of norepinephrine and serotonin to varying degrees depending on the agent. Although the efficacy of TCAs in the treatment of moderate and severe depression is well known, they have a number of adverse effects. The occurrence of dry mouth, constipation, urinary retention, and sedation may lead to noncompliance. More severe adverse effects, such as cardiac conduction delays and orthostatic hypotension, limit their use in the elderly. Furthermore, TCAs have a narrow therapeutic index, and overdosages can be life threatening. TCAs are the leading cause of hospital admissions for toxic ingestion (1).

The secondary amines, such as nortriptyline (Pamelor) and desipramine (Norpramin), are better tolerated than the tertiary amines, such as amitriptyline (Elavil) and imipramine (Tofranil). The secondary amines cause less orthostatic hypotension and fewer anticholinergic effects. The advantage of nortriptyline is that it has a therapeutic range of blood levels that can be used to achieve the most effective dosage.

Monoamine oxidase inhibitors. MAOIs (e.g., phenelzine [Nardil], tranylcypromine [Parnate]) are irreversible inhibitors of the enzyme monoamine oxidase and affect primarily the α-adrenergic system. They are effective in the treatment of combined depression and anxiety and are particularly useful in the treatment of atypical depression. When taking an MAOI, patients must avoid foods containing tyramine, such as certain cheeses and red wine, because the tyramine cannot be metabolized. Hypertension and, rarely, cerebral hemorrhage or death may ensue (9). MAOIs also have potentially fatal drug interactions with vasoconstrictors, decongestants, meperidine, and dextromethorphan (1). Short-acting reversible MAOIs may become available and would make this class of antidepressant more tolerable for patients and physicians.

Benzodiazepines. Benzodiazepines are sometimes prescribed for symptomatic relief in depressed patients. Unfortunately, these agents are sometimes given in lieu of antidepressants, and continued long-term use may result in habituation. Long-term use may also cause secondary depression. Benzodiazepine use should be restricted to low-dose, brief courses in patients who have concomitant anxiety and depression, and they should be terminated when antidepressants appear to be taking effect. Patients who have a history of substance abuse should not take them.

Treatment Guidelines

Acute phase. Successful treatment of depression requires careful follow-up. Patients with more severe depressions should be seen weekly for the first 6–8 weeks of acute treatment. Patients with less severe illness may be seen every 10–14 days for the first 6–8 weeks. Clinical improvement usually takes a minimum of 3–4 weeks to appear. Sleep and appetite disturbances typically improve before subjective mood experience improves. Once the depression has resolved, visits every 4–12 weeks are reasonable (17).

Office visits are essential in providing patient support and education and in monitoring clinical response. The key to increasing compliance is counseling the patient on the nature of depression, treatment options, potential medication side effects, and the importance of active participation in decision making and follow-through (1). By educating the patient's family (with the patient's permission), the practitioner may increase the likelihood of success. Frequent office visits facilitate medication dosage adjustments, if necessary, either to minimize side effects (because tolerance to the side effects has not occurred) or to improve response.

Maintenance phase. Patients who recovered from an initial or prior depressive episode at least 5 years earlier should be continued on the same antidepressant dosage for 6 months to 1 year after symptom remission is achieved. This practice reduced relapse rates by more than 50% during this time period compared with placebo (9). Patients with prior depressive episodes occurring less than 3 years earlier probably should be maintained on antidepressants at full dosage for 3–5 years. Patients with frequent recurrent depressive episodes may require lifetime treatment with antidepressants.

If a TCA is stopped suddenly, the patient may experience vomiting, diarrhea, headaches, sleep disturbances, or agitation. These symptoms may last for 1 month (25). Similar symptoms may occur with the cessation of the newer medications, more frequently with paroxetine, fluvoxamine, and venlafaxine than with fluoxetine or sertraline (25). Tapering of antidepressants over a 4-week period is recommended, but the taper rate should be based on the patient's tolerance of the taper (26).

Treatment Resistance

Despite the effectiveness of antidepressant medications, a significant proportion of depressed patients (10%–30%) do not respond to treatment (9). Failure to respond to an adequate medication trial is defined as no symptomatic improvement after 4 weeks of treatment, minimal early response that returns to baseline depression severity by week 5, or minimal improvement by week 6 (7, 26). Once treatment resistance has been identified, the diagnosis and the treatment need to be reassessed (7). Ongoing but undisclosed substance abuse or underlying general medical conditions may contribute to the lack of treatment response. If either factor is present, treatment should focus on the relevant potential cause. In cases of substance abuse, a 30-day substance-free state is usually sufficient to determine whether the depressive syndrome will remit without additional treatment. In cases of severe symptom presentations, the substance abuse and depressive disorders may require simultaneous treatment.

Several treatment options are available to augment response in patients with refractory depression. These options include maximizing the trial of the same antidepressant, changing to a different antidepressant, selecting a drug combination, or using a nonpharmacological treatment such as ECT. The most practical solution is to increase the dosage of the current antidepressant medication. Fluoxetine can be increased up to 40 mg/day or, in more severe cases, up to 60 mg/day or even 80 mg/day. Sertraline can be increased in 50-mg increments to 200 mg/day. Paroxetine can be increased in 10-mg increments to 50 mg/day. The practitioner should allow at least 1 week between dosage adjustments.

Medication combination trials usually involve augmentation of the current antidepressant with lithium carbonate, thyroid hormone, or stimulants (e.g., methylphenidate). Clinical data most strongly support the use of lithium. With regard to changing antidepressants, clinical data do not support the practice of switching from one SSRI to another when the first one fails. It is much more effective to change antidepressant class (24).

ECT is an extremely effective form of treatment for depression. Between 50% and 60% of patients who have failed to respond to a medication trial will respond to ECT (3). ECT is indicated particularly in patients with severe disease requiring rapid resolution of symptoms (e.g., in suicidal patients) and in patients with psychotic depression. The treatment is safe, even in medically compromised and elderly patients. Referral to a psychiatrist is required.

Nonpharmacological Treatment

Clinical outcome is generally improved when antidepressant treatment and psychotherapy are combined (1). Insight-oriented, supportive therapy and cognitive-behavioral therapy should be performed by a mental health professional; however, aspects of these therapies are part of any work with patients. The most important aspect is the maintenance of the doctor-patient relationship, which is therapeutic in and of itself. Primary care practitioners should play an active role in providing advice, reassurance, and problem solving. Patients should be encouraged to discuss psychological and social problems that result from chronic medical or psychiatric illnesses.

■ SPECIAL CLINICAL SITUATIONS

Geriatric Patients

Depression in the geriatric population (i.e., in those over age 65) is underdiagnosed and undertreated because signs and symptoms of depression often are interpreted as part of an irreversible dementing disorder or as a normal component of the aging process. The presentation is often insidious: depressed mood is less prominent than are changes in appetite or sleep, loss of interest, anergia, and social withdrawal. Depressed patients can also exhibit cognitive changes, known as *pseudodementia* or *dementia of depression.*

Most antidepressants are believed to be equally efficacious for geriatric depression. The risk of adverse drug effects is increased in the elderly because of the greater likelihood of comorbid medical disorders, the use of additional medications with potential drug interactions, and changes in metabolism (9). The SSRIs are effective for elderly patients, and these drugs, like all antidepressants, should be initiated at low dosages and the dosages increased slowly as needed. The shorter half-lives of sertraline and paroxetine may make these medications more appropriate for use than fluoxetine. If pseudodementia is suspected, a trial of an antidepressant may be worthwhile even if the diagnosis of depression versus dementia remains unclear (1). Patients with coexisting depression and dementia benefit from treatment of their depression (14). Methylphenidate has been used clinically as an adjunct to antidepressants (although it is not used with MAOIs) in treating some medically ill, apathetic, and withdrawn elderly patients. Because methylphenidate has a short half-life, it takes effect quickly and is used for several weeks until the antidepressant becomes effective. Methylphenidate is reported to have less cardiotoxicity than the TCAs. If the patient does not respond to 10–30 mg daily, then the methylphenidate should be stopped. Studies have not consistently demonstrated the efficacy of methylphenidate (20).

Suicidal Patients

One of the most important responsibilities primary care practitioners have for all depressed patients is to assess their risk for suicide. All patients with a depressed mood should be asked whether they have considered suicide or whether they have a history of suicide attempts. Patients should be questioned regarding the strength of the suicidal ideation or attempts and the lethality of the method contemplated. Patients may express a passive death wish (e.g., saying, "life is not worth living") without having true suicidal intent. Asking specific questions about suicide does not increase the likelihood of suicide or plant the idea in the patient's mind. The risk factors for suicidality are discussed in Chapter 11. Patients with suicidality should be referred to a psychiatrist as soon as possible.

■ CONCLUSION

Patients with mood disorders are commonly seen in primary care practices. The symptoms of depression, such as fatigue and weight loss, are often difficult to distinguish from those of chronic medical illnesses. Antidepressants and psychotherapy are effective forms of treatment. Patients who have severe depression, suicidality, or bipolar disorder should be referred to a psychiatrist before medications are started.

■ REFERENCES

1. Salazar WH: Management of depression in the outpatient office. Med Clin North Am 80:431–455, 1996
2. Kuzel R: Management of depression: current trends in primary care. Postgrad Med 99:179–195, 1996
3. American Psychiatric Association: Diagnostic and Statistical Manual of Mental Disorders, 4th Edition. Washington, DC, American Psychiatric Association, 1994
4. Wise MG, Rundell JR: Concise Guide to Consultation Psychiatry, 2nd Edition. Washington, DC, American Psychiatric Press, 1994

5. Katon W, Schulberg H: Epidemiology of depression in primary care. Gen Hosp Psychiatry 14:237–247, 1992
6. Greenberg PE, Stiglin LE, Finkelstein SN, et al: The economic burden of depression in 1990. J Clin Psychiatry 54:405–418, 1993
7. Depression Guideline Panel: Depression in Primary Care, Vol 2: Treatment of Major Depression. Clinical Practice Guideline No. 5 (AHCPR Publ No 93-0551). Rockville, MD, U.S. Department of Health and Human Services, Public Health Service, Agency for Health Care Policy and Research, 1993
8. El-Mallakh RS, Wright JC, Breen KJ, et al: Clues to depression in primary care practice. Postgrad Med 100:85–96, 1996
9. Charney DS, Miller HL, Licinio J, et al: Treatment of depression, in The American Psychiatric Press Textbook of Psychopharmacology. Edited by Schatzberg AF, Nemeroff CB. Washington, DC, American Psychiatric Press, 1995, pp 575–601
10. Mueller TI, Leon AC: Recovery, chronicity, and levels of psychopathology in major depression. Psychiatr Clin North Am 19:85–101, 1996
11. Depression Guideline Panel: Depression in Primary Care, Vol 1: Detection and Diagnosis. Clinical Practice Guideline No. 5 (AHCPR Publ No 93-0550). Rockville, MD, U.S. Department of Health and Human Services, Public Health Service, Agency for Health Care Policy and Research, 1993
12. Coyne JC, Schwenk TL, Fechner-Bates S: Non-detection of depression by primary care physicians reconsidered. Gen Hosp Psychiatry 17:3–12, 1995
13. Sturm R, Wells KB: How can care for depression become more cost-effective? JAMA 273:51–58, 1995
14. Williams-Russo P: Barriers to diagnosis and treatment of depression in primary care settings. Am J Geriatr Psychiatry 4 (suppl 1):84–90, 1996
15. Mulrow CD, Williams JW, Gerety MB, et al: Case-finding instruments for depression in primary care settings. Ann Intern Med 122:913–921, 1995
16. Elkin I, Shea MT, Watkins JT, et al: National Institute of Mental Health Treatment of Depression Collaborative Research Program: general effectiveness of treatments. Arch Gen Psychiatry 46:971–982, 1989
17. Katon W, Von Korff M, Lin E, et al: Adequacy and duration of antidepressant treatment in primary care. Med Care 30:67–76, 1992

18. Simon GE, Von Korff M, Wagner EH, et al: Patterns of antidepressant use in community practice. Gen Hosp Psychiatry 15:399–408, 1993
19. Schatzberg AF, Cole JO, DeBattista C: Manual of Clinical Psychopharmacology, 3rd Edition. Washington, DC, American Psychiatric Press, 1997
20. Hyman SE, Arana GW, Rosenbaum JF: Handbook of Psychiatric Drug Therapy, 3rd Edition. Boston, MA, Little, Brown, 1995
21. Bowden CL, Schatzberg AF, Rosenbaum A, et al: Fluoxetine and desipramine in major depressive disorder. J Clin Psychopharmacol 13:305–311, 1993
22. Nemeroff CB, DeVane CL, Pollock BG: Newer antidepressants and the cytochrome P450 system. Am J Psychiatry 153:311–320, 1996
23. Gardner EA, Johnston JA: Bupropion: an antidepressant without sexual pathophysiological action. J Clin Psychopharmacol 5:24–29, 1985
24. Preskorn SH: Selection of an antidepressant: mirtazepine. J Clin Psychiatry 58 (suppl 6):3–8, 1997
25. Zajecka J, Tracy KA, Mitchell S: Discontinuation symptoms after treatment with serotonin reuptake inhibitors: a literature review. J Clin Psychiatry 58:291–297, 1997
26. Quitkin F, McGrath PJ, Stewart JW, et al: Chronological milestones to guide drug change: when should clinicians switch antidepressants? Arch Gen Psychiatry 53:785–792, 1996

2

ANXIETY DISORDERS

Nitin Kulkarni, M.D.
Richard J. Ross, M.D.

Anxiety is a common emotional state. DSM-IV defines anxiety as "the apprehensive anticipation of future danger or misfortune accompanied by a feeling of dysphoria or somatic symptoms of tension" (1 [p. 764]). Anxiety has physiological and psychological manifestations. Its focus may be on perceived internal or external dangers. An anxiety disorder occurs when the symptoms are so intense that they cause personal distress or interfere with a person's daily functioning.

In a recent survey of the adult population, anxiety disorders ranked as the single largest mental health problem in the United States, with a 1-month prevalence of 17.2% (2). These disorders are diagnosed more commonly in young people (3). Between 14% and 66% of patients seen in a primary care setting have these illnesses (4). When an anxiety disorder occurs along with a medical disorder, such as hypertension or diabetes, greater overall impairment may be predicted (5). Even subthreshold symptoms of anxiety, which fail to meet the criteria for any syndrome, can cause significant disability in a primary care population (6). For these reasons, anxiety disorders must be recognized and treated promptly.

Correctly diagnosing an anxiety disorder may present a challenge to the primary care practitioner. For example, certain symptoms are shared by different anxiety disorders and hence are not pathognomonic of any one disorder. Also, patients with other mental disorders may experience pathological anxiety. Only if the anxiety symptoms can be viewed as independent would an additional diagnosis of an anxiety disorder be warranted.

■ SPECIFIC ANXIETY DISORDERS

In this chapter, we discuss the salient clinical features and the treatment of the anxiety disorders. Table 2–1 summarizes the essential characteristics of each of the anxiety disorders (1).

Panic Disorder

A panic attack is a discrete psychophysiological event involving extreme fear or discomfort. The onset is precipitous, and the symptoms build rapidly to a crescendo, generally within 10 minutes. A person in the throes of a panic attack may fear that something terrible is about to happen, that self-control is lost, or even that death is imminent. Patients may experience derealization (i.e., the feeling that the world is not real) and depersonalization (i.e. the feeling that one is detached from oneself). The somatic symptoms that occur during a panic attack are palpitations, diaphoresis, tremulousness, respiratory distress, nausea, abdominal discomfort, dizziness, and paresthesia.

The presence of recurrent, unexpected panic attacks is the sine qua non of panic disorder (1). The diagnostic criteria for panic disorder also require that the patient has, over at least 1 month, displayed concern about having another attack (so-called anticipatory anxiety), worried about the significance or consequences of the attacks, or showed a change in behavior related to the attacks (1). The psychosocial morbidity associated with panic disorder can be substantial. When severe restriction of outdoor activities occurs, the diagnosis of panic disorder with agoraphobia should be made.

Up to two-thirds of patients with panic disorder report symptoms during waking hours and during the non–rapid eye movement stage of sleep (7). Nocturnal or sleep panic attacks are associated with intense physiological arousal, sudden awakening, and terror. The patient may recall the details of the attack and may be unable

TABLE 2–1. **Characteristic symptoms of the anxiety disorders**

Disorder	Characteristic symptoms
Panic disorder	Discrete period of intense fear or discomfort
	Somatic symptoms (palpitations, diaphoresis, trembling) accompany attacks
	Concerns about recurrence of attacks (anticipatory anxiety)
Agoraphobia	Public places are feared and avoided because escape from such places is perceived to be difficult or because a panic attack may occur there
Social phobia	Fear of social or performance situations (may be manifested as panic attacks)
Obsessive-compulsive disorder	Presence of obsessions (recurrent, persistent, and intrusive thoughts or images) and/or
	Presence of compulsions (repetitive behaviors); for example, washing or counting performed to decrease anxiety or to prevent dreaded consequences
Posttraumatic stress disorder (PTSD)	Exposure to a traumatic event
	Trauma is reexperienced as flashbacks, nightmares, or intrusive thoughts
	Avoidance of people, places, or activities that serve as reminders of the trauma
	Hypervigilance, excessive startle response
Acute stress disorder	Exposure to a traumatic event
	Symptoms similar to PTSD but lasting only 2 days to 4 weeks
Generalized anxiety disorder	Excessive worry for at least 6 months
	Associated symptoms present (fatigue, sleep disturbance, muscle tension)
	Anxiety does not occur in discrete periods

(continued)

TABLE 2–1. **Characteristic symptoms of the anxiety disorders *(continued)***

Disorder	Characteristic symptoms
Anxiety disorder due to a general medical condition	Anxiety, panic, obsessions, or compulsions precipitated by a medical condition
Substance-induced anxiety disorder	Anxiety, panic, obsessions, or compulsions precipitated by intoxication with or withdrawal from a substance or medication

to return to sleep. Nocturnal panic attacks should not be confused with night terrors, which are usually preceded by a scream and followed by nearly total amnesia the morning after the event.

It is easy to see how some patients with panic disorder, feeling threatened by a perceived undiagnosed, serious illness and failing to accept the reassurance of caregivers that no medical illness exists, might repeatedly present to clinical offices and the emergency room. These patients quite often are labeled hypochondriacs, somatizers, or malingerers; however, in working with such patients, the practitioner must exclude medical conditions that can appear with panic-like symptoms.

The lifetime prevalence of panic disorder is 3.5%, and the female-to-male ratio is 2.5:1 (2). The age at onset varies, ranging from childhood to the 50s. A bimodal age distribution appears to exist, with peaks during adolescence and in the mid-30s. As with other anxiety disorders, this illness generally follows a chronic course (8); however, in the elderly, panic disorder is relatively uncommon (3).

Phobias

DSM-IV defines a phobia as "a persistent, irrational fear of a specific object, activity or situation (the phobic stimulus) that results in a compelling desire to avoid it" (1 [p. 770]). For the person with agoraphobia, situations from which escape would be difficult or embarrassing provide the phobic stimulus. When agoraphobia occurs together with panic disorder, the anxiety revolves around the possibility of having a panic attack while alone and helpless or trapped in a crowd. Alternatively, when agoraphobia occurs without a history of panic disorder, the anxiety is centered on the potential for some incapacitating or embarrassing event, though not a full-blown panic attack. If anxiety is focused on a certain object or situation—for example, on a particular type of animal or exposure to blood—the diagnosis of specific phobia is made. Although some anxiety is normal before a social engagement or before speaking in public, the patient with social phobia (or social anxiety disorder) may in such situations feel the object of intense scrutiny, about to be undone by the fear of humiliation or embarrassment. Patients with specific phobia and social phobia commonly experience panic symptoms said to be bound to the phobic stimulus; that is, they occur with a greater likelihood in its presence.

Any of the phobic disorders can severely compromise a person's everyday functioning. The agoraphobic individual, afraid to leave home, may be unable to report to work regularly or to shop for household necessities. People with a specific phobia—for example, of riding in an elevator—may avoid common activities. The person with social phobia may become uncomfortable even with seemingly simple tasks, such as asking for directions when lost, introducing oneself to others, or signing one's name. Associated physical discomfort may be present, including blushing, a sensation of "knots" in one's stomach, and an urgency to urinate.

Social phobia may be confused with agoraphobia; however, the socially phobic person primarily fears humiliation in meeting people, whereas the agoraphobic person essentially dreads the outside world but feels reassured if he or she can turn to someone for help. At times, it may be difficult to distinguish various personality disorders, especially avoidant personality disorder, from social phobia. An individual with schizoid personality disorder professes disinterest in socialization, whereas the socially phobic individual maintains an interest in human interactions.

The lifetime prevalence of social phobia is the highest (about 13%) among the anxiety disorders, followed by specific phobias and agoraphobia. Although the specific phobias and agoraphobia are about twice as common in females, social phobia has comparable lifetime prevalences in males and females (2). Unfortunately, only a minority of patients who have a phobic disorder seek professional help. The average age at onset is earlier for specific phobias (6–12 years) than for social phobia (adolescence) or agoraphobia (in the 20s). Phobias remain a fairly common disorder in the older age group; agoraphobia may be the only anxiety disorder with some likelihood of beginning in late life (3).

Obsessive-Compulsive Disorder

Obsessive-compulsive disorder (OCD) is characterized by obsessions, which are recurrent, unbidden distressing images or thoughts. An obsession might, for example, involve a concern over becoming contaminated or doing something violent. To control the resultant anxiety, obsessions are often followed by compulsions, which are repetitive behaviors (e.g., hand washing) and mental acts (e.g., counting) meant to combat the troublesome idea. The relief is temporary, however, and compulsions, too, feel distressing as they evolve into repetitive learned behavior. Although obsessions and compulsions wax and wane, they become time and energy consuming, and the person with OCD typically develops a repertoire of phobic avoidant behaviors. Resulting changes in lifestyle can lead to sometimes quite marked social and occupational impairment.

During the course of OCD, the individual generally recognizes the obsessions and compulsions as unreasonable and excessive. However, if his or her understanding of the symptoms becomes delusional, the prognosis is poor (9). Occasionally, isolated obsessions or compulsions may be present (in up to 15% of patients with OCD), although as many as one-half to two-thirds of patients show multiple obsessions and compulsions.

The diagnosis of OCD is sometimes missed because the practitioner may not have inquired into the symptoms or the patient may have concealed them. The lifetime prevalence of OCD is 2.5% and is equal in men and women. OCD commences in early adulthood, often in the 20s, with an earlier onset in men than in women. In the geriatric population, the prevalence decreases gradually with age.

Obsessive-compulsive personality disorder is different from and independent of OCD. It is characterized by rigidity and perfectionism that interferes with the completion of tasks, but it is not as distressing as OCD.

Generalized Anxiety Disorder

The cardinal feature of generalized anxiety disorder (GAD) is an uncontrollable tendency to become unduly worried over a range of issues, including those at school and at work. The source of anxiety can be as seemingly trivial as packing for an upcoming vacation or having one's routine upset by a brief power failure. It may seem difficult at times to differentiate normal worries from those seen in GAD; however, in GAD, the anxiety is pervasive and uncontrollable. The patient may experience insomnia, restlessness, edginess, irritability, and tension.

GAD exhibits a lifetime prevalence of 5%, with a male-to-female ratio of 1:2 (2). The average age at onset has been difficult to determine because when questioned, individuals with GAD commonly respond, "I've always been like this." In a geriatric sample exhibiting a 6-month prevalence of about 2%, fewer than 3% of cases began after age 65 (10). GAD tends to be even more chronic and unrelenting than panic disorder, although the attendant psychosocial disability may be less serious (8).

Adjustment and Stress Disorders

It may become clear in speaking with an anxious patient that the psychological distress relates specifically to an identifiable event or situation. A person experiencing a psychosocial stressor—such as difficulty in an interpersonal relationship, a financial setback, or an exacerbation of a chronic medical illness—may become uncharacteristically, excessively anxious and may, as a consequence, have impaired social or occupational functioning. When a temporal relationship between the stressor and such an emotional disturbance can be discerned, the patient may be said to have an adjustment disorder with anxiety. Although estimates of prevalence vary, adjustment disorder is not uncommon, particularly among people with unfavorable life circumstances.

When severe psychosocial stressors entail emotional trauma, a unique psychobiological response distinct from the adjustment disorder often ensues. A traumatic stressor is defined in DSM-IV as one in which the person "experienced, witnessed, or was confronted with an event or events that involved actual or threatened death or serious injury, or a threat to the physical integrity of self or others" and had a response involving "intense fear, helplessness, or horror" (1 [pp. 427–428]). Such stressors are exemplified by combat exposure, rape, or involvement in a natural disaster such as an earthquake. Some people describe a tendency to continually re-experience the trauma by imagining it, thinking or dreaming about it, or actually feeling as if it were recurring, in the form of a flash-back. At the same time, reminders of the trauma may be avoided, to the point that the individual disengages from normal activities and relationships, the so-called numbing response. Finally, some type of hyperarousal—perhaps an inability to fall or stay asleep, a low threshold for becoming angry, or a hypersensitivity to abrupt, loud noises— may be present. In the context of a severe stressor, the aforementioned triad of symptoms should suggest the diagnosis of a stress disorder.

A stress disorder that begins within 1 month of the traumatic experience and lasts no longer than 1 month is called an acute stress disorder. In contrast, a stress disorder that persists for longer than 1 month and takes an increasingly severe toll on a person's social and occupational functioning is called posttraumatic stress disorder (PTSD). Although PTSD frequently arises shortly after the occurrence of the traumatic stressor, it may have a delayed onset, appearing with no clear precipitant, as in the case of a well-adjusted, highly functional, asymptomatic veteran who, many years after the combat experience, suddenly becomes preoccupied with disturbing memories. PTSD did not enter formally into the nomenclature of mental disorders until 1980, but it is now generally agreed that the disorder has a high prevalence, affecting 1%–8% of the population over the course of a lifetime. PTSD seems to occur more frequently in women (11).

Anxiety Disorder Due to a General Medical Condition

If the presence of a medical disorder can account for the symptoms of any of the anxiety disorders, a diagnosis of anxiety disorder due to a general medical condition is made. This diagnosis rests at the confluence of psychiatric and medical disorders. Illnesses associated with prominent anxiety include neurological disorders (e.g., complex partial seizures, delirium, stroke); cardiovascular disorders (e.g., valvular disease, congestive heart failure, coronary artery disease, cardiac arrhythmias); pulmonary disorders (e.g., chronic obstructive pulmonary disease); and endocrinological disorders (e.g., hyperthyroidism, pheochromocytoma). The results of a comprehensive history and physical examination, along with routine laboratory tests and thyroid function tests, must be entered into the formulation of a differential diagnosis for symptoms of anxiety.

Substance-Induced Anxiety Disorders

When prominent symptoms of anxiety are thought to be the direct consequence of a substance, the diagnosis of substance-induced anxiety disorder is made. Syndromes that mimic primary panic attacks, phobias, OCD, and GAD can be seen in this disorder. A substance-induced anxiety disorder can occur in the context of either intoxication with or withdrawal from a substance such as alcohol, cocaine, amphetamines, cannabis, or hallucinogens. Withdrawal from alcohol, cocaine, benzodiazepines, and other sedative-hypnotic drugs can produce an anxiety disorder, with the latency of onset determined by the half-life of the offending substance. For example, because diazepam (Valium) has a long-lived metabolite, anxiety may not become a problem until 3 or more weeks into the period of abstinence. In contrast, because alprazolam (Xanax) has a short half-life, withdrawal symptoms such as anxiety may occur several hours after stopping the medication.

The use and abuse of prescription medications (e.g., theophylline), over-the-counter medications (e.g., those containing ephedrine), and certain herbal supplements can cause an anxiety disorder, and use of these substances needs to be explored in the patient's history. Caffeine in high doses is anxiogenic even in normal individuals, and it may precipitate frank panic attacks in patients who have panic disorder (12). In geriatric patients, the incidence of substance-induced anxiety disorders (e.g., panic attacks associated with alcohol abuse) is much lower than in younger adults, an observation that may relate to biological changes associated with aging such as degeneration in the brain's anxiogenic pathways (13).

■ COMORBIDITY

The presence of an anxiety disorder should alert the primary care practitioner to the possibility of coexisting mental disorders. For example, major depression may coexist with panic disorder, and substance abuse may worsen the course of PTSD. In general, the presence of undetected and untreated comorbid conditions exacerbates anxiety disorders and complicates their treatment. These conditions also may mask an underlying anxiety disorder. For example, alcohol withdrawal symptoms may make it difficult to identify underlying panic disorder. The risk of suicidal behavior may rise when panic disorder occurs with other psychiatric disorders; for example, the already high incidence of suicide attempts in panic disorder increases about fourfold in the presence of comorbidity (14).

The lifetime prevalence of major depression is 40%–70% in patients with panic disorder (15, 16) and is at least as high in patients with OCD (17). It may be difficult to separate the symptoms of an anxiety disorder from those of major depression. The restlessness of GAD may resemble the increased psychomotor activity of agitated depression. Consequently, a separate diagnostic entity called mixed anxiety-depressive disorder has been proposed.

In the Epidemiologic Catchment Area study of the National Institute of Mental Health, nearly one-quarter of the subjects with any anxiety disorder over their lifetimes also had a history of one or more substance abuse or dependence disorders, 1.7 times the prevalence in the general population (18). Panic disorder and OCD had particularly prominent associations with substance abuse or dependence. A recent national survey showed PTSD to have a high comorbidity with alcohol and drug abuse and dependence (11). The mechanisms underlying these reported associations require further research. Evidence suggests that anxiety disorders can precede the onset of substance abuse problems, in which case the patients may be seen as attempting to self-medicate their anxiety. In contrast, substance abuse has sometimes been viewed as a cause of anxiety disorders.

■ TREATMENT

Arrival at a proper diagnosis for symptoms of anxiety has significant implications for treatment. When anxiety occurs only in the context of a major mood disturbance, the latter should be treated with antidepressant and/or mood-stabilizing agents, and an antianxiety drug may be used adjunctively for symptomatic relief. When anxiety accompanies a psychotic episode in schizophrenia, an antipsychotic drug must be used, but an antianxiety agent used concomitantly may limit agitation. The anxious confusion of delirium is managed best by eliminating any reversible causes of central nervous system dysfunction and by judiciously instituting a low dosage of a high-potency antipsychotic drug. An antianxiety agent may provide relief, but the resulting inhibition of higher cortical function may further compromise already impaired consciousness-controlling mechanisms. The anxiety that accompanies dementia sometimes responds to an antianxiety agent, but again, the medication could worsen the confusion.

Any successful model of the treatment of anxiety disorders must encompass a biopsychosocial perspective of the patient. The clinician must attend to contributory medical problems, correctly diagnose the mental disorder(s), prescribe appropriate medications, and identify existing social stressors. In many cases, the primary care practitioner will be able to carry out these functions. Here we focus on the psychopharmacological interventions most likely to be used in the primary care setting.

Because treatment of the anxiety disorders is complicated, it is probably best to consider using a selective serotonin reuptake inhibitor (SSRI) and, if necessary, a benzodiazepine as initial pharmacological agents. Monoamine oxidase inhibitors (MAOIs), tricyclic antidepressants (TCAs), and augmenting strategies can be used only with psychiatric consultation. The expertise of a psychiatrist or another mental health professional should also be sought when the patient exhibits maladaptive personality traits or interpersonal relationships. Table 2–2 lists the medications used to treat anxiety disorders (19).

If a patient with an anxiety disorder has an active substance abuse or dependence problem, the problem must be identified and treated concurrently. The management of such dual-diagnosis patients presents complexities, and referral to a specialized treatment program should be made.

Panic Disorder

The SSRIs, which have good efficacy and a generally safe side-effect profile, have become the first-line drugs to treat panic disorder (20). The benzodiazepines are used effectively as a bridge until the SSRIs take effect, typically in 2–4 weeks. Table 2–3 lists the benzodiazepines commonly used to treat anxiety disorders (19). The short-term use of a benzodiazepine may alleviate some of the transient, anxiety-related side effects of the SSRIs (e.g., the *jitteriness syndrome*) (21). Once the therapeutic effect of an SSRI is observed, a benzodiazepine may also be used on an as-needed basis for breakthrough panic attacks. The TCAs imipramine and clomipramine are effective in treating panic disorder, but the likelihood of side effects and the potential for cardiovascular and other toxicities, particularly in overdosages, make them second-line agents. A meta-analysis comparing the SSRIs, the TCAs, and the benzodiazepines found the SSRIs to be superior to both imipramine and the benzodiazepine alprazolam (22). MAOIs provide another therapeutic alternative (see later in this chapter for special prescribing considerations).

The dosages for the individual SSRIs vary: for paroxetine (Paxil), the range is 10–60 mg/day, with higher dosages (40–60 mg/day) possibly having greater efficacy in reducing the frequency of panic attacks; fluvoxamine (Luvox) has been used in

TABLE 2–2. **Medications used to treat anxiety disorders**

Medication	Class	Dosage[a]	Indication(s)
Fluoxetine (Prozac)	SSRI	Initial dosage, 5–10 mg/day; therapeutic dosage, 20 mg/day; 40–80 mg/day for OCD	Panic disorder, OCD, PTSD, social phobia
Fluvoxamine (Luvox)	SSRI	Initial dosage, 50 mg/day; therapeutic dosage, 100–300 mg/day	OCD, PTSD, social phobia
Paroxetine (Paxil)	SSRI	Initial dosage, 10 mg/day; therapeutic dosage, 40–60 mg/day	Same as fluoxetine
Sertraline (Zoloft)	SSRI	Initial dosage, 25–50 mg/day; therapeutic dosage, 100–200 mg/day	Same as fluoxetine
Imipramine (Tofranil)	TCA	Initial dosage, 25–50 mg/day; therapeutic dosage, 150–300 mg/day	Panic disorder, GAD
Clomipramine (Anafranil)	TCA	Initial dosage, 25 mg/day; therapeutic dosage, 100–250 mg/day	OCD
Phenelzine (Nardil); tranylcypromine (Parnate)	MAOI	See text	Panic disorder, social phobia
Buspirone (BuSpar)	Nonbenzo-diazepine anxiolytic	Initial dosage, 5 mg/day bid; therapeutic dosage, 20–40 mg/day[b]	GAD
Propranolol (Inderal)	β-blocker	10–40 mg/day given 30 minutes prior to performance	Social phobia (performance anxiety)

Note. GAD = generalized anxiety disorder; MAOI = monoamine oxidase inhibitor; OCD = obsessive-compulsive disorder; PTSD = posttraumatic stress disorder; SSRI = selective serotonin reuptake inhibitor; TCA = tricyclic antidepressant.

[a]For geriatric patients, the initial dosage should be half of that listed; for these patients, the therapeutic dosage may also be lower.

[b]Supplied in a DIVIDOSE design such that tablets can be broken into halves (7.5 mg) or into thirds (5 mg).

TABLE 2–3. **Benzodiazepines commonly used to treat anxiety disorders**

Medication	Potency	Half-life (hours)	Therapeutic dosage (mg/day)[a]	Indication(s)
Diazepam (Valium)	Low	40–60	10–40[b]	GAD
Lorazepam (Ativan)	High	14	1–6	GAD
Oxazepam (Serax)	Low	9	30–60	GAD
Alprazolam (Xanax)	High	14	1–4[c]	GAD, panic disorder
Clonazepam (Klonopin)	High	18–50	1–3	GAD, panic disorder
Chlordiazepoxide (Librium)	Low	20–30	15–40	GAD

Note. GAD = generalized anxiety disorder. [a]Diazepam and clonazepam should be used on a bid or tid basis; the others can be given either tid or qid. [b]For geriatric patients, use half of the recommended dosages. [c]Initiate with 1.5 mg/day in divided dosages. May need 4–5 mg/day to treat panic disorder.

dosages up to 300 mg/day; for sertraline (Zoloft), the dosage range is 50–200 mg/day; and fluoxetine (Prozac) has been used at a dosage range of 5–80 mg/day. Higher dosages of the SSRIs may cause more side effects—typically gastrointestinal upset, nervousness, insomnia, and sexual dysfunction—and a higher dropout rate. The dosage at which the patient responds should be continued as maintenance treatment, in view of the fact that panic disorder is often chronic; only a subgroup of patients remain symptom free after discontinuing pharmacotherapy (8). Emerging evidence indicates that cognitive-behavioral therapy combined with antidepressant medication may offer an advantage over pharmacotherapy alone (23).

Specific Phobia

Cognitive-behavioral therapy often benefits patients who have a specific phobia (23). Cognitive distortions underlying the phobic response are addressed, and repeated exposure to the phobic stimulus, either imaginal or in vivo, in the secure setting of the clinical office, promotes desensitization. Medications may be considered if situational panic attacks are present (see preceding section and Table 2–2).

Social Phobia

The MAOI phenelzine (Nardil) (45–75 mg/day) has well-established efficacy in treating social phobia (24). Awareness of the dietary restrictions on tyramine-containing foods (e.g., certain cheeses; red wines, Chianti, and dark beers; soy sauce), is critical, as is knowledge of potential side effects (e.g., orthostatic hypotension, sexual dysfunction) and of potentially dangerous drug interactions (e.g., with any sympathomimetic agent; with TCAs, SSRIs, or other antidepressants; or with the opiate drugs meperidine and dextromethorphan). Patients must be cautioned not to take even an over-the-counter cold remedy without first consulting the primary care practitioner, and they should be reminded to advise their dentists, who might otherwise use epinephrine as a vasoconstrictor mixed with a local anesthetic. Once the maximum benefit is realized, the MAOI should be continued for at least 6 months before a decision is made to taper and then stop the medication.

The rate of relapse after discontinuing pharmacotherapy can be decreased by combining cognitive-behavioral therapy with medication (25). The SSRIs also appear to have a role in treating social phobia (26). Given the relative safety of the SSRIs compared with MAOIs, some clinicians recommend SSRIs as first-line agents (27). When the risk of psychological dependence is judged not to be high and comorbid depression is not present, a benzodiazepine such as clonazepam (Klonopin) may be preferred over an antidepressant (28). Of the β-blockers, propranolol (Inderal) (10–40 mg on an as-needed basis) may diminish the symptoms of sympathetic arousal in the subtype of social phobia that is performance related (i.e., performance anxiety).

Obsessive-Compulsive Disorder

As discussed earlier, a dysfunction of the serotonergic system has been implicated in OCD; perhaps not surprisingly, the SSRIs have become the mainstay of treatment, although typically the dosages required are higher than those used in major depression, and the time required to see a beneficial effect is longer (8–10 weeks). Clomipramine (Anafranil), a TCA with attendant anticholinergic and other side effects, is also commonly used. If the patient does not respond to an SSRI after an adequate dosage has been tried for a sufficient time, clomipramine may be used; likewise, an SSRI can serve as an alternate drug if clomipramine was prescribed first without success. The MAOIs phenelzine and tranylcypromine (Parnate) may be used in treating refractory OCD (29), but the appropriate washout period is required after discontinuing TCAs and other antidepressants (at least 2 weeks, but 5 weeks for fluoxetine) to prevent dangerous drug interactions such as the serotonergic syndrome and hypertensive crisis. A drug is said to have failed after it has been tried at the maximum dosage for 10–12 weeks. The maximum daily dosages are 60 mg for paroxetine, 80 mg for fluoxetine, 200 mg for sertraline, 300 mg for fluvoxamine, and 250 mg for clomipramine.

When partial benefits are observed, an augmentation strategy can be used before abandoning an SSRI or clomipramine trial. Augmentation can involve the use of buspirone (BuSpar, an agonist for the serotonin$_{1A}$ receptor), lithium, or clonazepam. Given the risk of tardive dyskinesia, neuroleptics are to be used with caution to treat OCD; indications include the presence of delusional obsessions and comorbid conditions such as Tourette syndrome. OCD typically is chronic. Lifelong medication may be required; otherwise, relapse may occur after the discontinuation of treatment. A psychosocial treatment called *exposure and response prevention,* wherein obsessional thoughts are provoked in patients while ritualistic thoughts and behaviors are prevented, has demonstrated efficacy in the long-term management of OCD (23).

Generalized Anxiety Disorder

The benzodiazepines have long been the first-line treatment for flare-ups of anxiety in GAD. Although many benzodiazepines are available in the United States, long-acting drugs such as diazepam have been preferred to shorter-acting agents such as alprazolam, which carry a higher risk of anxiety rebound between doses (30). Dosages of diazepam in the range of 10–40 mg/day typically suffice. The drug may accumulate over time, however, and troublesome side effects may emerge. This situation creates a problem particularly in the elderly and in those with cirrhosis, who often have a reduced metabolizing capacity. If a benzodiazepine is to be used in these individuals, oxazepam (Serax) or lorazepam (Ativan), both of which depend on glucuronidation alone for elimination, should be considered. The benzodiazepines may also be categorized by their potency, or the amount of the drug necessary to produce a clinical effect. High-potency benzodiazepines produce more severe withdrawal symptoms (19). Clonazepam and alprazolam have a high potency, whereas oxazepam has a low potency (31).

The benzodiazepines can lead to physical dependence, which could emerge as early as 3–4 months into treatment, and the discontinuation of even low doses can lead to withdrawal reactions (8). Despite the typical chronicity of GAD, strategies for maintenance therapy have not been well delineated. Many patients will require prolonged treatment in order to avoid recurrences, and the benzodiazepines retain their efficacy at least 6 months into a course of treatment (32). Periodically, the practitioner should make an effort to taper the drug dosage for patients receiving maintenance treatment, but even with a gradual reduction, withdrawal symptoms may be expected, and these symptoms are often difficult to distinguish from a recurrence of the underlying anxiety disturbance (33).

For nonresponders or partial responders, a second agent such as the TCA imipramine (34) or the SSRI fluvoxamine (35) may be used. Buspirone is preferred by some psychiatrists for the treatment of GAD in patients who have a history of alcohol or sedative-hypnotic abuse. The drug, which should be started at 5 mg tid and increased as needed up to 20 mg tid, is nonsedating, has few side effects, and has no abuse potential.

Stress Disorders

Few studies have been conducted on the pharmacotherapy or psychotherapy of stress disorders. This situation is particularly surprising given the marked symptom overlap between PTSD and other anxiety disorders and the mood disorders, the majority of which are highly responsive to both pharmacotherapy and cognitive-behavioral treatments. The SSRIs, TCAs, and MAOIs can benefit some patients, but the symptoms of PTSD generally recur. Evidence, predominantly from work with rape victims, suggests that behavioral strategies that incorporate desensitization and relaxation training may retard or prevent the development of chronic PTSD (36).

CONCLUSION

The anxiety disorders have a high prevalence in the primary care population. They entail a high cost to patients in the form of intense personal, occupational, and social distress, regardless of whether the symptoms reach a syndromal threshold. They often are comorbid with, and difficult to distinguish from, other psychiatric illnesses. Newer insights into the neurochemistry and psychobiology of the anxiety disorders continue to yield useful tools in alleviating the many symptoms of anxiety.

REFERENCES

1. American Psychiatric Association: Diagnostic and Statistical Manual of Mental Disorders, 4th Edition. Washington, DC, American Psychiatric Association, 1994
2. Kessler RC, McGonagle KA, Zhao S, et al: Lifetime and 12-month prevalence of DSM-III-R psychiatric disorders in the United States. Arch Gen Psychiatry 51:8–19, 1994
3. Flint AJ: Epidemiology and comorbidity of anxiety disorders in the elderly. Am J Psychiatry 151:640–649, 1994
4. Sherbourne CD, Jackson CA, Meredith LS, et al: Prevalence of comorbid anxiety disorders in primary care outpatients. Arch Fam Med 5:27–35, 1996
5. Sherbourne CD, Wells KB, Meredith LS, et al: Comorbid anxiety disorder and the functioning and well being of chronically ill patients of general medical providers. Arch Gen Psychiatry 53:889–895, 1996
6. Olfson M, Broadhead E, Weissman MM, et al: Subthreshold psychiatric symptoms in a primary care group practice. Arch Gen Psychiatry 53:880–886, 1996
7. Mellman TA, Uhde TW: Sleep panic attacks: new clinical findings and theoretical implications. Am J Psychiatry 146:1204–1207, 1989
8. Schweizer E: Generalized anxiety disorder: longitudinal course and pharmacologic treatment. Psychiatr Clin North Am 18:843–853, 1995
9. Jenike MA, Baer L, Minichiello WE, et al: Coexistent obsessive-compulsive disorder and schizotypal personality disorder: a poor prognostic indicator (letter). Arch Gen Psychiatry 43:296, 1986

10. Blazer D, George LK, Hughes D: The epidemiology of anxiety disorders: an age comparison, in Anxiety in the Elderly: Treatment and Research. Edited by Salzman C, Lebowitz B. New York, Springer, 1991
11. Kessler RC, Sonnega A, Bromet E, et al: Posttraumatic stress disorder in the National Comorbidity Survey. Arch Gen Psychiatry 52:1048–1060, 1995
12. Charney DS, Heninger GR, Jatlow PI: Increased anxiogenic effects of caffeine in panic disorder. Arch Gen Psychiatry 42:233–243, 1985
13. Krystal JH, Leaf PJ, Bruce ML, et al: Effects of age and alcoholism on the prevalence of panic disorder. Acta Psychiatr Scand 85:77–82, 1992
14. Johnson J, Weissman MM, Klerman GL: Panic disorder, comorbidity, and suicide attempts. Arch Gen Psychiatry 47:805–808, 1990
15. Lesser IM: Panic disorder and depression: co-occurrence and treatment, in Clinical Aspects of Panic Disorder. Edited by Ballenger JC. New York, Wiley-Liss, 1990, pp 181–191
16. Lydiard RB: Coexisting depression and anxiety: special diagnostic and treatment issues. J Clin Psychiatry 52 (suppl 6):48–54, 1991
17. Rasmussen SA, Eisen JL: The epidemiology and clinical features of obsessive-compulsive disorder. Psychiatr Clin North Am 15:743–758, 1992
18. Regier DA, Farmer ME, Rae DS, et al: Comorbidity of mental disorders with alcohol and other drug abuse: results from the Epidemiologic Catchment Area (ECA) study. JAMA 264:2511–2518, 1990
19. Schatzberg AF, Cole JO, DeBattista C: Manual of Clinical Psychopharmacology, 3rd Edition. Washington, DC, American Psychiatric Press, 1997
20. Sheehan DV, Harnett-Sheehan K: The role of SSRIs in panic disorder. J Clin Psychiatry 57 (suppl 10):51–60, 1996
21. Pohl R, Yergani VK, Balon R, et al: The jitteriness syndrome in panic disorder patients treated with antidepressants. J Clin Psychiatry 49: 100–104, 1988
22. Boyer W: Serotonin uptake inhibitors are superior to imipramine and alprazolam in alleviating panic attacks: a meta-analysis. Int Clin Psychopharmacol 10:45–49, 1995
23. Barlow DH, Lehman CL: Advances in the psychosocial treatment of anxiety disorders. Arch Gen Psychiatry 53:727–735, 1996
24. Liebowitz MR, Schneier F, Campeas R, et al: Phenelzine vs. atenolol in social phobia: a placebo controlled comparison. Arch Gen Psychiatry 49:290–300, 1992

25. Liebowitz MR, Marshall RD: Pharmacological treatment of social phobia: clinical applications, in Social Phobia: Diagnosis, Assessment, and Treatment. Edited by Heimberg R. New York, Guilford, 1995, pp 366–386
26. Van Vliet I, den Boer JA, Westenberg HGM: Psychopharmacological treatment of social phobia: a double-blind, placebo-control study with fluvoxamine. Psychopharmacology 115:128–134, 1994
27. Marshall RD, Schneier FR: An algorithm for the pharmacotherapy of social phobia. Psychiatric Annals 26:210–216, 1996
28. Davidson JRT, Petts N, Richichi E, et al: Treatment of social phobia with clonazepam and placebo. J Clin Psychopharmacol 13:423–428, 1993
29. Jenike MA, Surman OS, Cassem NH, et al: Monoamine oxidase inhibitors in obsessive-compulsive disorder. J Clin Psychiatry 4:131–132, 1983
30. Hyman SE, Arana GW, Rosenbaum JF: Handbook of Psychiatric Drug Therapy, 3rd Edition. Boston, MA, Little, Brown, 1995
31. Salzman C: Anxiety in the elderly: treatment strategies. J Clin Psychiatry 51 (suppl):18–21, 1990
32. Rickels K, Case WG, Downing RW, et al: Long-term diazepam therapy and clinical outcome. JAMA 250:767–771, 1983
33. Schweizer E, Rickels K, Case WG, et al: Long-term therapeutic use of benzodiazepines. Arch Gen Psychiatry 47:908–915, 1990
34. Rickels K, Downing R, Schweizer E, et al: Antidepressants for the treatment of generalized anxiety disorder. Arch Gen Psychiatry 50: 884–895, 1993
35. Laws D, Asford JJ, Antee JA: A multicenter double blind comparative trial of fluvoxamine versus lorazepam in mixed anxiety and depression treated in general practice. Acta Psychiatr Scand 81:185–189, 1990
36. Rothbaum BO, Foa EB, Riggs DS, et al: A prospective examination of post-traumatic stress disorder in rape victims. J Trauma Stress 5:455–475, 1992

3

SUBSTANCE USE DISORDERS

Wayne Barber, M.D.

The motives for substance use are many: to alleviate distress, to dispel social awkwardness, to improve sexual satisfaction or performance, to enable a sense of belonging, or to experience pleasure. Whatever the rationale, such use can advance readily to abuse and dependence. Good clinical practice requires early identification and treatment of substance use disorders. Current economic necessity directs that such treatment occur on an outpatient basis whenever possible. In this chapter, I review the addictive states most commonly encountered in the office setting, offering guidelines for timely recognition, effective primary care, and referral for more specialized treatment.

■ GENERAL PRINCIPLES

DSM-IV lists seven criteria involved in making the diagnosis of substance dependence, also known as addiction (see Table 3–1) (1). Five criteria are behaviors; the other two are physiological phenomena. Although tolerance and withdrawal are frequently part of dependence, their presence alone does not enable the clinician to make the diagnosis. The essential part of the diagnosis involves one or more of the behavioral components listed in Table 3–1.

The term *substance abuse* refers to clinically significant use that, though maladaptive, falls short of addictive self-administration. This label helpfully identifies those patients whose use puts them

TABLE 3–1. **DSM-IV criteria for substance dependence**

The occurrence of three of the following seven criteria in the same 12-month period is sufficient for the diagnosis of substance dependence:

Behavioral patterns of compulsive use (recalled by the mnemonic *TEACH*):

(1) Inordinate **t**ime spent obtaining, using, or recovering from effects of the substance

(2) Consumption **e**xceeds amount intended (in quantity and/or duration of use)

(3) Patient's usual **a**ctivities are reduced or forsaken (work, family, play)

(4) Patient attempts to **c**ontrol and/or curtail use

(5) Despite awareness of **h**armful consequences, patient fails to limit use

Criteria for physical dependence:

(1) Tolerance: a reduction in effect occurring after repeated use of a substance, commonly resulting in increased self-administration, in an effort to renew the desired experience

(2) Withdrawal: a substance-specific rebound phenomenon following cessation or reduction of use, comprising physiological changes opposite in effect to those that produced the dependence

Source. Adapted from American Psychiatric Association 1994 (1).

at risk for dependence. Table 3–2 summarizes the criteria for substance abuse.

The onset of dependence is based on the pharmacokinetic properties of each specific agent and its route of administration, in concert with certain innate attributes of the host. The more rapid its onset of effect, or swift its withdrawal, the more likely a substance will continue to be used. This situation can be complicated further by any additional factors that extend the duration of withdrawal, which then portend a greater likelihood of relapse.

Some patients will not admit their substance abuse. Instead, they will seek treatment for medical or psychological problems. Thoughtful history taking on the practitioner's part is required to

TABLE 3–2. **DSM-IV criteria for substance abuse**

The occurrence of any of the following criteria in the same 12-month period is sufficient for the diagnosis of substance abuse (recalled by the mnemonic CLOD):

- Adverse **c**onsequences in social/interpersonal sphere fail to deter continued use
- Recurring problems in **l**egal area related to substance use
- Failure to meet major role **o**bligations because of recurrent substance use
- Recurrent substance use occurs in **d**angerous circumstances (such as driving or operating heavy machinery)

Source. Adapted from American Psychiatric Association 1994 (1).

discover those interpersonal, financial, legal, and work-related difficulties that could point to the presence of a substance use disorder. It is often helpful to obtain additional history (with the patient's consent) from other sources regarding the patient's quality of life at home, at work, and within his or her community. It is particularly important to ask about the individual's use of other agents because dependent individuals often use more than one substance.

An addictive illness often generates a clinical picture indistinguishable from those of other major psychiatric illnesses, differentiated only by its prompt remission with abstinence. Correspondingly, substance use disorders commonly coexist with other psychiatric illnesses. As a result, it can be difficult to determine the source of psychiatric symptoms in the setting of active substance use or to predict the course of those symptoms. The practitioner is well advised to make thoughtful observations of the patient's behavior and perform a thorough mental status examination in anticipation of future comparison. As always, acute emotional states merit prompt attention. The practitioner must be especially watchful for indications that the patient's behavior might pose a danger to him- or herself or others; however, initiation of long-term treatment of chronic conditions such as psychosis or depression should be avoided until drug or alcohol effects have been stabilized and the course of the illness has been clarified.

■ GENERAL GUIDELINES FOR TREATMENT

To be successful, rehabilitation must address every relevant area of the patient's personal and family difficulties. Because physiological dependence may lead to withdrawal when the substance is discontinued, the practitioner must be prepared to offer detoxification specific to the agent of abuse. I describe techniques specific to the various substances of abuse later in this chapter.

Although detoxification from physical dependence is commonly a necessary first step toward recovery, it does not provide enduring benefit, nor does it improve outcome on its own. The factor most predictive of long-term success is the duration of rehabilitation treatment, with 2 years as the watershed for persisting change. Effective rehabilitation is best provided by specialized facilities with the following critical attributes:

- Therapeutic milieu with other recovering addicts
- Skilled staff adept at managing manipulative behaviors
- Specialized counseling emphasizing relapse prevention

Although most substance-dependent individuals respond well to skilled outpatient treatment, practitioners must correctly identify those individuals needing inpatient care and refer them appropriately. Four general conditions necessitate hospital treatment:

1. Inability to discontinue use despite adequate outpatient treatment
2. Presence of medical or psychiatric conditions warranting close observation (e.g., Wernicke-Korsakoff syndrome, delirium tremens (DTs), risk of seizure, active psychosis, homicidal or suicidal risk)
3. Inadequate psychosocial support system (e.g., homelessness, disorganized living situation, caregivers of compromised judgment)
4. Need to interrupt a living situation that strongly reinforces continued use (e.g., caregivers who help perpetuate the patient's use of substances or substance-using family members)

Practitioners should become aware of local resources that can provide necessary comprehensive services. Evidence indicates that successful addiction treatment depends on a breadth of services that match the specific needs of individual patients. Fortunately, patients who meet the criteria for comprehensive outpatient programs do equally well as inpatients, as long as equivalent treatment services are offered. Particular concern should be directed toward the treatment given individuals who have concomitant psychiatric diagnoses to ensure they receive appropriate psychiatric treatment.

Most patients are ambivalent about starting treatment interventions. Once the diagnosis has been made, the clinician should share with the patient the findings that indicate a substance use problem, using clear and unequivocal language and a tone of acceptance and understanding. In an effort to help the patient recognize that he or she has a substance use disorder, it is sometimes effective to explain that the patient's past medical difficulties, psychological problems, marital discord, or occupational dysfunction may be the consequences of substance use.

■ SPECIFIC SUBSTANCES AND TREATMENT

Tables 3–3 and 3–4 summarize the signs and symptoms of intoxication with and withdrawal from the substances discussed in this chapter.

Alcohol

Presentation. Although most alcoholic individuals never seek treatment, they appear frequently at the primary care practitioner's office. A flushed face, slurred speech, a garrulous manner, and ataxia each strongly suggest the possibility of alcoholic intoxication. Problem drinking may be suspected if the patient has a poorly explained accident or injury, especially in the presence of current confusion. A history of recent blackouts frequently can be obtained. Unexplained hypertension is often due to alcoholism. Physical findings of chronic liver disease, acute gastritis, dehydra-

TABLE 3–3. **Signs and symptoms of intoxication**

	Alcohol, benzodiazepines, barbiturates	Cocaine, other stimulants	Opiates	Marijuana
Signs				
Eyes	Nystagmus; miosis when severe	Mydriasis (may necessitate sunglasses)	Miosis is prominent	Injected conjunctivae
Vital signs	Stage dependent; chronic use increases blood pressure	Heart rate and blood pressure usually increase, although may decrease; varied arrhythmia	Bradycardia, risk of respiratory depression; pulmonary edema	Tachycardia
Neuromotor	Incoordination to unsteady gait, slurred speech	Dyskinesia, dystonia, muscle weakness, seizures	Slurred speech	Impaired coordination
Psychomotor	Agitation, combativeness	Agitation (sometimes retardation); stereotyped behaviors	Activity is usually outside normal range; may be increased or decreased	Passive
Sensorium	Impaired concentration and memory; stupor to coma	Confusion to coma	Impaired attention and memory; drowsiness to coma	Impaired attention, memory, and sense of time
Autonomic	Diaphoresis, flushed face and skin	Diaphoresis, chills	—	Dry mouth

Gastro-intestinal/nutrition	Poor nutrition	Nausea, vomiting, marked weight loss, poor nutrition	Constipation, poor nutrition	Increased appetite
Integument and mucosa	Dental neglect	Needle marks and tracks, ulcerated nasal septum, dental neglect	Needle marks and tracks, dental neglect	—
Symptoms[a]				
Mood	Labile	Euphoria to blunting; anxiety, tension, or anger	Euphoria to apathy; or dysphoria	Euphoria and/or anxiety
Judgment	Impaired	Impaired	Impaired; sensation of slowed time	Impaired
Social and occupational functioning	Impaired	Impaired	Impaired	Social withdrawal

Note. [a]*Symptoms* are defined as clinically significant maladaptive behaviors or psychological changes that developed during or shortly after use.
Source. Adapted from Barber and O'Brien 1995 (2).

TABLE 3–4. **Signs and symptoms of withdrawal**

	Alcohol, benzodiazepines, barbiturates	Cocaine, other stimulants	Opiates	Marijuana
Signs				
Eyes	—	—	Mydriasis	Photophobia
Vital signs	Heart rate > 100 beats/minute, increased blood pressure and temperature	—	Fever, increased heart rate and blood pressure	Tachycardia
Neuromotor	Hand tremor, seizures	—	—	Tremors
Psychomotor	Agitation	Agitation or retardation	Irritability, restlessness	Restlessness, irritability
Sensorium	Transient hallucinations	Vivid and/or unpleasant dreams	—	Confusion
Autonomic	Diaphoresis	—	Diaphoresis, yawning, lacrimation, rhinorrhea, piloerection, chills	Chills, diaphoresis, yawning
Gastrointestinal/nutrition	Nausea or vomiting	Increased appetite	Vomiting, diarrhea	Nausea, diarrhea, anorexia, weight loss
Mood	Anxiety	Dysphoria	Dysphoria	Anxiety, depression

Sleep	Insomnia	Insomnia or hypersomnia	Insomnia	Insomnia
General	Fatigue	Myalgia	Fatigue, myalgia	Myalgia

Source. Adapted from Barber and O'Brien 1995 (2).

tion, or peripheral neuropathy oblige the practitioner to explore further. Evidence pointing to acute pancreatitis or esophageal varices requires an aggressive inquiry into the patient's history of alcohol use. Intense confusion in association with hallucinosis warns of the possible approach of DTs or Wernicke-Korsakoff syndrome, both life-threatening conditions.

Laboratory studies. No single test is sufficiently sensitive or specific to substantiate the diagnosis, but several clusters of laboratory results implicate alcohol dependence. A substantial elevation in γ-glutamyl transferase (GGT) levels associated with increased mean corpuscular volume (MCV) is highly suggestive of heavy alcohol intake. Certain changes in the liver function tests are pathognomonic of hepatic injury produced by ethanol (see Table 3–5). In the absence of obvious signs of intoxication, a blood alcohol content (BAC) greater than 150 mg/dL is diagnostic of alcoholism (3).

Elevation of levels of carbohydrate deficient transferrin (CDT), an iron transport protein affected by heavily sustained ethanol intake, is now commonly interpreted as evidence of recent excessive drinking. Renewed elevations in GGT or CDT levels once abstinence has been sustained over several weeks indicate the patient has started drinking again (4). Table 3–5 summarizes these and other laboratory abnormalities (3).

Good patient care depends on specific diagnostic studies to assess the medical consequences of alcohol abuse. In addition to a routine complete blood count and urinalysis, liver function tests, prothrombin test, and albumin, electrolyte, glucose, calcium, and magnesium levels should be obtained. For patients over age 40, an electrocardiogram is recommended. The BAC is an uncomplicated office determination that aids diagnosis and enables more specific treatment for those needing detoxification. Because alcoholic individuals often concurrently abuse other drugs, a urine drug screen should be ordered whenever available.

Drug interactions. The effects of alcohol on the liver and the brain can be problematic with the concurrent use of certain

TABLE 3–5. **Abnormal findings in heavy users of alcohol**

Measure	Percentage of heavy users showing increase in this measure
Carbohydrate deficient transferrin (CDT)	80
γ-glutamyl transferase (GGT)	67
Aspartate transferase (AST)	50
Alanine transferase (ALT)	50
Mean corpuscular volume (MCV)	25
Triglycerides	25
Alkaline phosphatase (AP)	17
Bilirubin	14
Uric acid	10
Markers of alcoholic liver injury	
AST:ALT > 2	
GGT:AP > 3.5	

medications, generating adverse effects during both chronic use and withdrawal. The greatest jeopardy stems from alteration of liver enzyme systems and enhancement of respiratory depression. For example, the use of acetaminophen is contraindicated in the setting of excessive alcohol intake and its consequent liver injury (5). Table 3–6 lists the effects of alcohol on the metabolism of other commonly used medications.

Withdrawal. In most cases, withdrawal can be managed in the practitioner's office. The findings are tremors, autonomic hyperactivity, gastrointestinal distress, sleep disturbance, and anxiety. Patients with concurrent illnesses, such as chronic obstructive pulmonary disease (COPD), and those who abuse other substances, such as benzodiazepines, may have more severe withdrawal symptoms and may warrant vigilant monitoring.

Detoxification. Medicated detoxification is warranted when the withdrawal symptoms are more than mild. The minimization

TABLE 3–6. **Interactions between alcohol and common medications**

Medication	Effect of alcohol on blood level	Other effects
Barbiturates	Increases	With combined use, risk of fatal respiratory depression
Benzodiazepines	Increases	Inhibits first-pass metabolism after oral ingestion
Phenothiazines	Increases	Competitive inhibition of hepatic metabolism
Phenytoin	Decreases	Enzyme induction increases clearance
Opiates	Increases	Mutually potentiating
Acetaminophen	Increases	Alcohol increases hepatotoxicity

of physical and psychic distress safeguards against a return to drinking while reducing the risk of serious medical complications. Daily office visits are required in order to monitor the patient's vital signs and BAC, assess his or her mental status, and provide support. It is imperative that a sober, stable family member or friend assist the patient with this home-based procedure.

Because chronic drinking reduces an individual's ability to absorb thiamine, replacement should be provided (100 mg/day po) for the first 10 days as protection against the emergence of Wernicke-Korsakoff syndrome. Parenteral administration may be required for several days in patients reluctant to accept oral treatment. Because the patient's nutrition has usually been compromised, multivitamins are suggested for the first month.

In most circumstances, benzodiazepines are the drugs of choice for detoxification. Although many practitioners favor the convenience of longer-acting preparations, the practitioner should be aware of the greater safety and flexibility offered by short-acting compounds, such as oxazepam (Serax) and lorazepam (Ativan), which have minimal abuse potential and little risk of accumulation, given the absence of active metabolites. The initial dose should be large enough to relieve withdrawal symptoms and should then be tapered gradually over 5–7 days. An initial dosage of oxazepam 30–60 mg qid is usually sufficient, supplemented by 15–30 mg every 6 hours as needed for breakthrough insomnia, shakes, nausea, vomiting, or anxiety. The medication is then reduced 15–30 mg/day as symptoms permit, with the diminishing dosage spaced evenly throughout the day. Lorazepam, which offers the additional benefit of being available for intramuscular and intravenous administration, may be used in a similar schedule with an equivalency of 1 mg for each 15 mg of oxazepam. Table 3–7 summarizes the medications used in the treatment of alcohol and other forms of substance abuse (6, 7).

Because withdrawal can be prompted by any decrease in blood level, symptoms may appear even while alcohol is significantly present in the bloodstream. The practitioner should avoid undermedicating the patient, because doing so increases the risk of seizures or a return to drinking. It is equally important to resist the premature use of benzodiazepines, which in combination with alcohol might induce respiratory depression.

Fever greater than 101°F, delirium, severe autonomic hyperactivity, fluctuating levels of cognitive efficiency, or hallucinations herald the onset of DTs and require immediate attention. Wernicke's encephalopathy should be suspected when global confusion and cerebellar ataxia are noted and is certain when ophthalmoplegia is also present. These conditions are life-threatening medical emergencies (8). Because the risk of suicide is high in patients with alcoholism, its likelihood must be assessed carefully.

Rehabilitation. Studies show that without further treatment after detoxification is completed, patients quickly return to drinking. The best outcomes are achieved through comprehensive programs offering patient education, relapse prevention strategies, training in new coping skills, employment counseling, an emphasis on alcohol-free social and recreational activities, and the active support of family and an abstinent community such as Alcoholics Anonymous. Research has demonstrated that day hospital treat-

TABLE 3–7. **Medications used to treat substance abuse**

Medication	Indication(s)	Dosage and administration
Oxazepam (Serax)	Alcohol, benzodiazepine detoxification	30–60 mg/day in divided doses, supplement with 15–30 mg every 6 hours as needed, titrate toward withdrawal symptoms, reduce dosage 15–30 mg/day over 5–7 days
Disulfiram (Antabuse)	Maintenance of abstinence from alcohol	> 170 pounds, use 250 mg/day; < 170 pounds, use 125 mg/day
Naltrexone (Trexan)	Maintenance of abstinence from alcohol (decreases craving)	50 mg/day
Nicotine polacrilex (Nicorette gum)	Nicotine replacement	2-mg dose per hour as needed,[a] wean one dose per week after 1–2 months of treatment
Transdermal nicotine (Nicotine patch)	Nicotine replacement	If patient smokes more than 10 cigarettes/day, start with highest dose available (15–22 mg, depending on brand); after 1–2 months, taper using the lower dosages for 2–4 weeks each
Nicotine nasal spray (Nicotrol NS)	Nicotine replacement	One or two sprays to each nostril, use hourly as needed, do not use more than 40 mg/day, use for 8 weeks and then taper over 4 weeks
Bupropion (Zyban)	Smoking cessation	150 mg in morning for 3 days, then 150 mg bid for 7–12 weeks

Alprazolam (Xanax)	Alprazolam detoxification	If patient is taking 3–5 mg/day, decrease 0.5 mg/day every 5–7 days to 2 mg/day, then decrease 0.25 mg/day every 7 days
Clonazepam (Klonopin)	Alprazolam detoxification	Substitute clonazepam at half of dosage of alprazolam; adjust dosage of clonazepam for sedation or withdrawal symptoms
Clonidine (Catapres)	Opiate detoxification	0.1–0.2 mg every 8 hours for 2–3 days,[b] can use 0.2–0.4 mg every 8 hours if withdrawal symptoms persist, taper by 25%–33% every day
Phenobarbital/ pentobarbital	Barbiturate, benzodiazepine, alcohol detoxification	Give pentobarbital 100–200 mg every 6 hours,[c] then convert to phenobarbital[d]; give phenobarbital every 8 hours for 2 days, then decrease dosage by 30 mg/day until taper is complete

Note. [a]Heavy smokers should start with a 4-mg dose. [b]Do not use clonidine if systolic blood pressure is less than 90 mm Hg. [c]Heavy users may require 300–500 mg of pentobarbital every 6 hours. [d]100 mg pentobarbital = 30 mg phenobarbital.

ment comprising these elements is as effective as inpatient care, at a fraction of the cost (9). Well-timed interventions based on motivation to change enhance outcome greatly. Outcome studies indicate that the patient's length of time in treatment best predicts sustained recovery. In the current era of managed care, outpatient programs are proliferating as inpatient services become much less available. When available, day hospital treatment comprising a comprehensive range of services is preferred.

Pharmacotherapy. Because in even the most effective treatment programs half the patients relapse within 3 months, there has been an intensive search for medications that could improve outcome. For many years, disulfiram (Antabuse) was the only medication available to impede an individual's return to drinking. It was used for its aversive physiological interaction with ethanol. Through inhibition of the enzymatic activity of acetaldehyde dehydrogenase, treatment with disulfiram leads to the toxic accumulation of acetaldehyde in proportion to the quantity of alcohol ingested, yielding a range of unpleasant symptoms including tachycardia, flushing, shortness of breath, nausea, and vomiting. The side effects of disulfiram include fatigue and a metallic taste. Early in treatment, a fatal hepatitis may occur; for this reason, liver function tests need to be conducted prior to initiation of treatment and 2 weeks after treatment has begun (6). Problems with compliance have limited the usefulness of disulfiram to only the most motivated of patients (10).

More recently, research has been concentrated on the inhibition of craving and reinforcement. Naltrexone, an opioid antagonist, currently offers the greatest promise. The opioid compensation hypothesis proposes that alcohol stimulates the production of endogenous endorphins, which evoke dopaminergic stimulation of the reward center, the nucleus accumbens. In blocking this sequence at the μ receptor, naltrexone significantly reduces alcoholic euphoria, craving, and the number of days spent drinking, while cutting in half the risk of slips proceeding to full relapse. The recommended regimen is 50 mg po daily for at least 6 months. This treatment is effective only with the compliant patient who is also engaged in a relapse prevention program. Given conflicting data regarding the effect of naltrexone on liver function, it should be used cautiously in patients with elevated bilirubin levels or substantially increased levels of liver enzymes. Other common side effects include nausea, vomiting, insomnia, headache, and nervousness (6). The practitioner should carefully inquire about recent opiate use to avoid precipitating acute opiate withdrawal.

Nicotine

Tobacco smoking prevails as the leading preventable cause of illness and death in the United States. More than 400,000 deaths yearly are attributable to smoking, nearly one-fifth of the nation's total (11). Addiction to nicotine maintains smoking behaviors. Most smokers claim they want to stop, and in any given year, one-third of them try. Yet less than one-fourth of those who try to stop succeed in their first attempt. Almost two-thirds fail to finish the first week. Rapid respiratory delivery promptly induces pharmacological dependence, and the discomfort of withdrawal closely follows each cigarette. Meanwhile, those highly developed habit patterns associated with smoking are intensely reinforced by the reward center, the nucleus accumbens, thus conditioning their persistence.

Presentation. It is no longer uncommon for patients to ask their primary care practitioner for help with smoking cessation. Usually they have already tried several times to stop on their own. The practitioner may be alerted by the presence of shortness of breath; chronic, productive cough; bronchial asthma; or COPD. When encountering evidence of hypertension, chronic cardiac disease, peripheral vascular disease, or peptic ulcer, the practitioner should ask the patient whether he or she smokes.

Withdrawal. Typically, symptoms begin within 12 hours of the last cigarette, peak within a few hours, and continue for several weeks. Craving, anxiety, irritability, restlessness, difficulty concentrating, diminished heart rate, and increased appetite are each noted in more than two-thirds of withdrawing subjects. Interrupted sleep accompanied by intense dreaming is common. Patients with a history of a psychiatric disorder are more prone to a mood disturbance during withdrawal (12).

Treatment. Most people find it difficult to stop smoking without help. The primary care practitioner is ideally positioned to identify smokers and address the dangers of their habit. The practitioner can capture the most cases by asking all patients whether they smoke and by taking a careful smoking history of those who do. Firm advice to stop, personalized to reflect an individual's specific risks, is usually well received. Patients motivated to quit smoking should be encouraged to set a quit date for the near future and be provided with self-help materials. A supportive phone call from the practitioner around the intended quit date significantly enhances success. Table 3–8 lists resources available for finding structured cessation programs.

Nicotine replacement is generally required by the highly dependent smoker, particularly when any of the following criteria are met:

- The individual smokes more than 10 cigarettes per day
- The individual seeks to smoke within 30 minutes of awakening

TABLE 3–8. **Resources for smoking cessation**

National Cancer Institute: (800) 4-CANCER
Helpful Pamphlets
Why Do I Smoke?
Clearing the Air
Quit for Good
American Cancer Society: (800) 227-2345
American Academy of Family Physicians: (800) 274-2237

- The individual's prior attempts to quit failed within the first week

A well-studied regimen with an established safety record offers nicotine patch replacement beginning with 21 mg/day, tapering over an 8-week period. If this program is less than optimal, individualization of dosage and duration may be considered, with adjustment made according to the patient's progress. Current research demonstrates a dose-response curve for the administration of nicotine that supports prescribing the patch according to the individual's characteristic smoking pattern. Containing the symptoms of withdrawal may require an initial dosage of 42 mg/day for heavy smokers (> 40 cigarettes/day) and 28–35mg/day for moderately heavy smokers (25–40 cigarettes/day).

Because patches are now available in a variety of strengths both by prescription and over the counter, they may be combined to achieve the desired dosage. It is best not to combine brands, because they differ in their rates of delivery. Heavier smokers, particularly those who struggle with intense cravings, may supplement their patch treatment with nicotine polacrilex chewing gum, every 2–4 hours at times of an irresistible desire to smoke. Because transmucosal absorption of nicotine requires a basic solution, patients should avoid drinking coffee, tea, or cola drinks close to the time they are using the gum. Because patients who fail to achieve abstinence within the first 2 weeks have a greatly reduced expectancy of success, practitioners should schedule a return visit within a 2-week period to reinforce the patient's effort.

Although not innocuous, nicotine administered in this manner presents minimal risk, far less than that associated with continued smoking. The practitioner should be alert for nicotine toxicity in patients with cardiac conditions, COPD, peptic ulcer, and peripheral vascular disease. Recently, a 2- to 3-month course of 300 mg/day of sustained-released bupropion (Zyban) has been suggested as a treatment for smoking cessation. Whether it is more effective than the patches is not known, but the long-term relapse rate is high with both bupropion and patches (13).

Studies demonstrate a relationship between smoking and recurrent major depression. Patients with a history of this disorder have much poorer outcomes, displaying greater difficulty in stopping and a tendency to relapse more readily. These individuals are also more vulnerable to an exacerbation of their depression on withdrawal from nicotine (14). The use of antidepressant medication for moderating withdrawal and reducing the risk of depression has been explored, and bupropion appears to be effective for both indications.

Outcome is enhanced greatly by providing structured, supportive counseling, including continuing education, praise and encouragement, and relapse prevention training (15). Appointments should be scheduled every 1–2 weeks while the patient is in the process of smoking cessation.

Benzodiazepines

Substances used to relieve anxiety are addicting. Similar problems are encountered with the benzodiazepines: swift pharmacological dependency, subtle cognitive deficits, blackouts, uncomfortable withdrawal, and questionably durable benefit. Although few patients exceed the therapeutic dosage range, many readily develop pharmacological dependence, some find the drug hard to relinquish, and a few escalate their use to the point of becoming addicted. Because primary care practitioners write the majority of prescriptions, it is particularly important that they be watchful for excessive use and supportively intervene to assist in tapered withdrawal for those patients displaying a pattern of abuse. Practitioners must be particularly cautious with the elderly, whose slower hepatic detoxification of these drugs and their metabolites puts them at risk for oversedation and physiological dependence. Moreover, because older patients are more likely to be taking other medications, practitioners must watch for problematic drug interactions.

Low-dose dependence. For the first several months of therapeutic dosing, mild rebound anxiety and insomnia may follow within several hours of the most recent dose. Patients who receive treatment for more than 4 months may be reluctant to go without. After 1 year of use, most patients will experience significant withdrawal on abrupt discontinuation of the drug. Even in the absence of behavioral patterns of compulsive use, this situation merits medically supervised detoxification.

Some patients are particularly vulnerable to the effects of these drugs. Those with chronic dysphoria and personality disorder are more prone to dependency and abuse. Abstinent alcoholic patients and those with a history of drug dependence are at serious risk (16).

High-dose dependence. Occasionally, a patient treated appropriately finds the drug so reinforcing that he or she increases the dosage without the physician's knowledge. More commonly, those addicted to other substances will use benzodiazepines adjunctively. Alcoholic patients take them both to augment their reward and to mute the pain of withdrawal. Street addicts seek them to assuage cocaine toxicity, ease opiate withdrawal, or boost the limited euphoric potential of methadone. Because it is hard to distinguish the effects of benzodiazepines from those of the primary drug of abuse, the practitioner should look for indications of benzodiazepine use whenever alcohol abuse or illicit drug use is encountered.

Specific notice should be taken regarding the ready development of physical dependence on alprazolam (Xanax). Its swift absorption and its rapid transit through the blood-brain barrier yield intense euphoria and the quick development of tolerance and dependence. As a result, escalation of use to high-dose dependence is relatively common. Accordingly, the use of this drug should be discouraged in favor of the many less-problematic benzodiazepines currently available (17).

Adverse effects. After prolonged use, most patients experience subtle memory problems and blackouts, of which they are often not aware. Some people become intoxicated at therapeutic dosage levels. Depression, anxiety, or hostility can be exacerbated, and social indiscretions as a result of impaired judgment or emotional lability may also occur. These effects are augmented greatly by the concomitant use of alcohol.

Withdrawal. The time until the appearance of symptoms varies greatly with the elimination half-life of each drug and its active metabolites. Because high-potency compounds with shorter half-lives (e.g., alprazolam, lorazepam) induce more immediate and intense discomfort, they are more commonly abused. In general, withdrawal symptoms are the opposite of what the benzodiazepines produce, namely central nervous system hyperarousal. The first symptoms to appear are profound rebound anxiety and insomnia accompanied by general restlessness. Tremors, sweating, weight loss, and myoclonus are often noted. Tachycardia, hypertension, and agitation may also occur. Inconsistently, patients may later develop a cluster of findings that are pathognomonic of benzodiazepine withdrawal: confusion, depersonalization, perceptual distortions, paresthesia, hyperacusis, and photophobia (16).

Though rare, seizures can occur during the early withdrawal period, typically within 3 days of discontinuation of drug use. Patients at risk for seizures during withdrawal have a history of high-dose dependence when taking a long-acting compound such as diazepam. Seizure risk is increased substantially by the concomitant use of other sedating agents, particularly alcohol.

Detoxification. The abrupt discontinuation of benzodiazepines is medically unsound. Most low-dose–dependent patients will experience some physical distress during withdrawal, and many will become apprehensive, anticipating discomfort without their medication. All patients should be informed regarding the need for discontinuation and should be trained in alternative ways of managing their distress. Because some patients may be actively drinking or using other psychotropic medication, a full history should be taken before benzodiazepines are tapered.

Withdrawal may be managed either by tapered administration

of the drug of use or by substitution of a longer-acting benzodiazepine, such as clonazepam or chlordiazepoxide, in an effort to level the receding dosage. Propranolol can assuage the symptoms of autonomic excitation. If, in the course of recovery, the patient displays an underlying panic disorder, depression, or phobia, the institution of specific therapy may then be appropriate. The antihypertensive clonidine and psychotropics (e.g., carbamazepine medications) are in general not effective and may pose problems in management.

Studies consistently report that the time of greatest challenge is the final period of tapered drug administration and the first abstinent week. A gradually extending taper is needed to minimize discomfort and to prevent the onset of withdrawal seizures or delirium. One study reported that an exponential reduction of 50% every 5 days not only avoided this terminal distress but also prevented the appearance of the protracted withdrawal syndrome (18). Some patients continue to experience waves of recurring symptoms for several months after the completion of the taper. These symptoms include anxiety, depression, tinnitus, paresthesia, formication, motor symptoms, and gastrointestinal complaints. Careful attention to the graduation of taper reduces the likelihood of onset of these symptoms.

Low-dose–dependent patients without medical complications or significant alcohol consumption may be treated on an outpatient basis. In contrast, those dependent on higher-than-therapeutic dosages or who are using benzodiazepines in combination with significant alcohol or other substances of abuse require a medicated detoxification that begins in the hospital.

Overdosages. Though rarely fatal, overdosages are commonly encountered in the emergency room in the context of a suicide gesture or attempt. Care should be taken to detect the concomitant ingestion of other sedatives, particularly alcohol, which greatly increase the risk of life-threatening respiratory depression. Flumazenil, a competitive benzodiazepine antagonist, may be given by intravenous infusion to interrupt this morbid effect.

Substances Encountered Occasionally in Primary Care Settings

Prescribed opiates. From time to time, the clinician will encounter in the office setting a patient whose pain management has led to dependent use. A patient may find opiate-induced relaxation and euphoria so appealing that he or she escalates his or her use in response to rapidly increasing tolerance, only to become trapped between abuse and the distress of withdrawal. Careful monitoring of patients' requests for prescription refills can avoid this situation. Once abuse is detected, the physician is obliged to advise the patient of his or her excessive use and the need for a tapered opiate withdrawal. Moreover, few patients will long tolerate the discomforts of short-acting opiate withdrawal before seeking another source for their prescriptions. Referral to a specialized clinical facility for structured methadone withdrawal or, when necessary, methadone maintenance is generally the better choice.

In the absence of a psychosocial pattern of drug dependence, patients who receive opiates for organically based pain uncommonly experience euphoria and rarely become opiate dependent. If treatment of pain is adequate, the practitioner should not let fear of addiction override the patient's need for analgesia. The physician must remain watchful for individuals seeking narcotic treatment for poorly explained pain symptoms. These patients may be managed with nonsteroidal anti-inflammatory drugs or referred to an available pain clinic for individualized treatment.

Cocaine. Since its successful chemical isolation first enabled potent bioavailability in 1859, cocaine's popularity has cycled. Because the street use of low-cost, smokable crack has escalated, snorting of the powder has declined markedly. Cocaine is often used with alcohol.

Cocaine abuse should be considered in patients exhibiting unexplained chronic rhinitis, unexplained bradycardia, or an ulcerated nasal septum. It should also be included in the differential diagnosis of patients who present with seizures, myocardial ischemia, cardiac arrhythmia, or psychosis (19). Recent withdrawal from use may be suspected in the context of depressed mood, irritability, and intense insomnia that fades to lethargy or apathetic depression, accompanied by urgent hunger and a prominent desire for sleep.

If the practitioner detects cocaine abuse, he or she should refer the patient for specialized treatment. Cocaine cravings can be so powerful that they readily prompt relapse. Long-term care may be needed, because brief treatments are generally ineffective. To date, no medications have proven useful in the management of this dependence.

Heroin. In recent years, the price of heroin has dropped significantly while its purity has increased sharply. Consequently, snorting and smoking of high-potency heroin are on the rise, occasionally presenting in the office setting in isolated local epidemics, especially among young people. Dependence may be indicated by the presence of withdrawal signs such as prominent mydriasis, lacrimation, rhinorrhea, yawning, pronounced autonomic arousal, or low-grade fever. The presence of needle tracks indicates intravenous self-administration. If the practitioner detects heroin dependence, he or she should refer the patient for supervised methadone withdrawal, because those who are exposed to unmedicated withdrawal are far less likely to remain in treatment.

Barbiturates. Once the sedative-hypnotics of popular choice, barbiturates are now less frequently encountered in the practitioner's office setting as primary drugs of abuse, although they may be seen as but one ingredient in polysubstance use. Patients seeking relief from pain may excessively self-administer butalbital (Fiorinal and related compounds). The low therapeutic index of barbiturates, their reinforcement at therapeutic dosages, and their cross-tolerance with both alcohol and benzodiazepines portend significant problems in management, warranting inpatient care. Respiratory depression and withdrawal seizures are the most significant dangers. Overdosages require intensive supportive care—in particular, the maintenance of adequate respiration.

Hallucinogens. Since 1990, hallucinogen use by young people has been on the rise. The temporary alteration of thought, perception, and mood that hallucinogens induce does not commonly prompt users to seek medical attention. Patients will occasionally present with complaints of panic anxiety as part of a "bad trip." Reassurance and a calm atmosphere usually are sufficient treatment, although low doses of benzodiazepines may be used to mute dysphoria. Phencyclidine (PCP) deserves special mention because its reinforcing qualities readily promote abuse, especially when it is rapidly administered by smoking. Use of PCP can cause a thought disorder, hallucinations, and assaultive behavior. PCP dosage-related anesthetic effects lead to stupor and coma in heavy abusers, accompanied by muscular rigidity, rhabdomyolysis, and hyperthermia (20). Early signs of intoxication in individuals who have a history of PCP use may warrant emergency care.

Marijuana. The use of marijuana (cannabis) has not demonstrated the severity of physical damage or dependence observed with other addicting substances, but evidence indicates that habitual use can be harmful. Tolerance and mild physical dependence are commonly encountered, yielding a withdrawal syndrome characterized by irritability, anxiety, restlessness, insomnia, anorexia, weight loss, chills, and tremors. Higher dosages can produce derealization, depersonalization, flashbacks, loss of insight, and even illusions or hallucinations. Alterations of mood, memory, motor coordination, and cognitive efficiency tend to persist long after the passing of desired pleasurable effects. Because few patients seek help for marijuana use alone, and such use produces nonspecific symptoms and signs, the detection of marijuana abuse is made through taking a careful history.

Interest has developed recently in the medicinal use of marijuana. The active ingredient of marijuana, delta-9-tetrahydrocannabinol (THC), is now available in a prescription medication, dronabinol. Dronabinol is effective in treating the nausea that develops as a side effect of cancer chemotherapy (21). It is also useful in the wasting syndrome of acquired immunodeficiency syndrome (AIDS) (21). THC also lowers intraocular pressure in glaucoma but needs to be taken continuously in order to be of benefit (21). There is no medical indication for smoking marijuana, especially because it exposes the patient to higher levels of carcinogens than does smoking tobacco. Also, bacteria have been cultured from marijuana, which means that immunosuppressed patients who use marijuana are at particular risk (21).

■ CONCLUSION

Substance abuse and dependence are commonly seen in primary care practices. When taking a patient's medical history, the practitioner should routinely ask questions about the extent of substance use. Treatment can be complicated and may require hospitalization and a referral to a specialist.

■ REFERENCES

1. American Psychiatric Association: Diagnostic and Statistical Manual of Mental Disorders, 4th Edition. Washington, DC, American Psychiatric Association, 1994
2. Barber WS, O'Brien CP: Addictions: early identification and intervention in an office setting. Primary Psychiatry 2:49–55, 1995
3. DuPont RL: Laboratory diagnosis, in Principles of Addiction Medicine. Edited by Miller NS. Chevy Chase, MD, American Society of Addiction Medicine, 1994
4. Litten RZ, Allen JP, Fertig JB: γ-Glutamyltranspeptidase and carbohydrate deficient transferrin: alternative measures of excessive alcohol consumption. Alcohol Clin Exp Res 19:1541–1546, 1995
5. MacDonald J, Twardon CM, Shatter HS: Alcohol, in Source Book of Substance Abuse and Addiction. Edited by Friedman LS, Fleming NF, Roberts DH, et al. Baltimore, MD, Williams & Wilkins, 1996, pp 109–137

6. Schatzberg AF, Cole JO, DeBattista C: Manual of Clinical Psychopharmacology, 3rd Edition. Washington, DC, American Psychiatric Press, 1997
7. Henningfield JE: Nicotine medications for smoking cessation. N Engl J Med 333:1196–1202, 1995
8. McMicken DB: Alcohol withdrawal syndromes. Emerg Med Clin North Am 8:805–819, 1990
9. Alterman AI, O'Brien CP, McLellan AT: Differential therapeutics for substance abuse, in Clinical Textbook of Addictive Disorders. Edited by Frances RJ, Miller SI. New York, Guilford, 1991, pp 369–390
10. Fuller RK, Branchey L, Brightwell DR, et al: Disulfiram treatment of alcoholism: a Veterans Administration cooperative study. JAMA 256: 1449–1455, 1986
11. Bartecchi CE, MacKenzie TD, Schrier RW: The human costs of tobacco use. N Engl J Med 330:907–912, 975–980, 1994
12. Haxby D: Treatment of nicotine dependence. Am J Health Syst Pharm 52:265–281, 1995
13. Bupropion (Zyban) for smoking cessation. Med Lett Drugs Ther 39:77–78, 1997
14. Glassman AH, Covey LS: Nicotine dependence and treatment, in Psychiatry. Edited by Michels R. Philadelphia, PA, Lippincott-Raven, 1996
15. Hughes JR: An overview of nicotine use disorders for alcohol/drug abuse clinicians. Am J Addict 5:262–274, 1996
16. Juergens SM: Benzodiazepines and addiction. Psychiatr Clin North Am 16:75–86, 1993
17. Juergens SM: Alprazolam and diazepam: addiction potential. J Subst Abuse Treat 8:43–51, 1991
18. Lader M, Morton S: Benzodiazepine problems. British Journal of Addiction 86:823–828, 1991
19. Mackler SA, O'Brien CP: Cocaine abuse. Adv Intern Med 37:21–35, 1991
20. Brendel D, West H, Hyman SE: Hallucinogens and phencyclidine, in Source Book of Substance Abuse and Addiction. Edited by Friedman LS, Fleming NF, Roberts DH, et al. Baltimore, MD, Williams & Wilkins, 1996, pp 217–229
21. Voth EA, Schwartz RH: Medical application of delta-9-tetrahydrocannabinol and marijuana. Ann Intern Med 126:791–798, 1997

4

COGNITIVE DISORDERS

Michael F. Gliatto, M.D.

Dementia is characterized by symptoms that affect intellectual performance. Memory loss is the most frequent complaint, but patients may demonstrate deficiencies in language; perception; praxis; or the ability to learn new skills, solve problems, think abstractly, and make judgments (1). These symptoms begin insidiously and worsen over time.

It is often difficult to distinguish between the beginning stages of dementia and the cognitive changes that occur in all people as they age. The hallmark of dementia, however, is that the cognitive changes interfere with the patient's daily responsibilities such as taking care of a house, paying bills, maintaining social relationships, or working (2).

Two to three million Americans are demented; by the year 2000, there may be five to six million (3). Between 40% and 60% of people in nursing homes are demented (3). Prevalence increases with age so that dementia affects 2%–3% of the population aged 65–79 but affects greater than 20% of the population older than 80 years (3).

Dementia has a number of possible causes. At autopsy, approximately 70% of patients with dementia exhibit the characteristic pathological changes associated with Alzheimer's disease. In 15% of patients with dementia, the dementia is from vascular causes, Pick's disease, or Lewy body disease. In the remaining 15%, more than one disease process is evident (4).

■ SPECIFIC DEMENTIAS

Although dementia is often classified as *potentially reversible* or *irreversible,* a completely reversible dementia is rare. Table 4–1 lists common causes of dementia.

Except for major depression, I do not discuss potentially reversible conditions in this chapter, although it should be noted that many medications may cause dementia. The most commonly cited are antihypertensives, sedative-hypnotics, psychotropics, anticonvulsants, cimetidine, and digitalis (5).

Alzheimer's Disease

Patients with Alzheimer's disease decline gradually. Memory loss is often the first symptom noticed by patients or their families, but patients can exhibit other initial symptoms, such as visuospatial problems, behavioral problems, or personality changes prior to the onset of memory loss (6).

The course of the decline is approximately 8–10 years. Patients initially need help with executive functions, such as paying bills or shopping, but as the disease advances, they require assistance with dressing, bathing, and using the toilet. In the final stages, patients become incontinent and immobile and they cannot speak (7). Death results from complications, such as poor nutrition, pneumonia, or aspiration. There are some forms of Alzheimer's disease with a strong genetic component in which patients present with symptoms in their late 40s or early 50s and the decline is rapid (3–5 years). In other forms of the disease, the decline may be much slower (15–20 years) than the usual course (8).

In Alzheimer's disease, morphological changes occur in parts of the brain, such as the hippocampus and the temporal lobe, that are associated with the regulation of memory, emotion, and behavior. These changes include cortical atrophy, neuronal loss, cytoplasmic neurofibrillary tangles, and neuritic plaques (which consist of β-amyloid, a neurotoxin) (1). Chemically, there is a reduction in the amount of acetylcholine, a neurotransmitter in-

TABLE 4–1. **Common causes of dementia**

Cause	Example	Course
Medications	See text	Potentially reversible
Endocrinological disorder	Hypothyroidism	Potentially reversible
Metabolic abnormality	Hyponatremia	Potentially reversible
Central nervous system infection	Neurosyphilis	Potentially reversible
	Human immunodeficiency virus	Irreversible
Brain lesions	Subdural hematoma	Potentially reversible
	Normal-pressure hydrocephalus	Potentially reversible
	Tumors	Potentially reversible
	Head trauma	Mostly irreversible
Nutritional deficiencies	Folate	Potentially reversible
	Vitamin B_{12}	Potentially reversible
Psychiatric disorders	Major depression	Reversible
	Alzheimer's disease	Irreversible
	Vascular dementia	Irreversible
	Parkinson's disease	Irreversible

volved in memory. This finding has treatment implications, as I discuss later in this chapter.

Risk factors for Alzheimer's disease include advanced age, a family history of the disease, and the apolipoprotein E (APOE)–4 allele of chromosome 19 (9). APOE is involved in cholesterol transport in the brain, and individuals who have the E4 allele have an increased risk of developing Alzheimer's disease by age 85 (10). Those with the E2 allele have a lower risk of developing the disease. Not everyone with the E4 allele develops dementia, and some patients with Alzheimer's disease do not have the E4 allele. Thus routine genetic screening is not recommended at this time (4, 9). One study found that patients with Alzheimer's disease had elevated cerebrospinal fluid levels of neural thread protein (11). This finding may have a role in clarifying the physiology of Alzheimer's disease and in the development of treatment for the disease.

Vascular Dementia

Vascular dementia has a stepwise or ratchet-like course of decline, in contrast to the gradual decline observed in Alzheimer's disease. A stepwise course is one in which there is a sudden decline in premorbid function that does not progress further until another precipitous change occurs some unpredictable time later. Dementia results once a certain amount of brain tissue, especially that vital to cognition, is infarcted. Risk factors for vascular dementia are those of cerebrovascular accidents—for example, hypertension, coronary artery disease, hypercholesterolemia, a history of smoking, and atrial fibrillation (10).

Subcortical Dementias

Some dementias are *subcortical,* in that they involve brain structures internal to the cerebral cortex. These dementias include those associated with Huntington's disease and Parkinson's disease. Huntington's disease is a genetic disorder that causes the degeneration of the caudate nucleus, resulting in chorea, dementia, and psychosis.

Parkinson's disease results from degeneration of the basal ganglia, causing rigidity, tremors, and gait abnormalities. The clinical distinction between Parkinson's disease and Alzheimer's disease can become blurred. Thirty percent of patients with Parkinson's disease develop dementia, either secondary to Alzheimer's disease or from another cause, and 30% of patients with Alzheimer's disease have rigidity or postural abnormalities (12). The dementia of Parkinson's disease has the same symptoms as that of Alzheimer's disease except that visual impairment is more pronounced (13). Diffuse Lewy body disease is a dementia in which Lewy bodies, usually seen in subcortical brain structures in patients with Parkinson's disease, are distributed widely in the cortex, usually in association with plaques and tangles. Patients with Lewy body disease exhibit dementia before the onset of extrapyramidal symptoms (14).

Dementia Secondary to Alcoholism

Alcoholic patients experience a variety of chronic cognitive symptoms. In Korsakoff's syndrome, a consequence of Wernicke's encephalopathy, the patient has anterograde and retrograde memory impairment, but other cognitive abilities, such as language, are spared (15). Patients who abuse alcohol over many years may develop dementia, wherein all cognitive capabilities are affected. The dementia may be a result of many factors, including direct neurotoxicity from alcohol, vitamin deficiencies, recurrent head trauma, and liver disease (15).

Other Irreversible Dementias

Rarer forms of dementia include Pick's disease and Creutzfeldt-Jakob disease. Pick's disease is one of the frontal lobe dementias. Frontal lobe dementias are associated with personality changes (which develop before cognitive symptoms), apathy, disinhibited behavior, and preserved praxis and visuospatial abilities (10, 12). In addition, patients with Pick's disease have language disturbances, such as excessive speech and repetition of words (12).

Creutzfeldt-Jakob disease is a dementia caused by proteinaceous infectious material known as *prions*. Sources of prions include infected growth hormone and corneal transplants. The dementia that results from infection by prions progresses over the course of 1–2 years and is associated with generalized myoclonus (12). Slowing and periodic complexes are seen on electroencephalograms (12).

■ EVALUATION

The key to the diagnosis of confusion and memory loss is a thorough history. Obtaining a good history may be difficult in that patients can minimize symptoms because they are embarrassed or are not aware of the problem. The family frequently initiates contact with the practitioner. It is best to take the history from the patient first, and then, in the patient's presence, take a second history from the family members or caregivers. The history should include an assessment of how the patient carries out the responsibilities of daily life. For instance, the practitioner should ask how the patient prepares meals, cleans the house, dresses, bathes, shops, drives, or pays bills. A gradual deterioration in the performance of these skills suggests dementia.

The evaluation should include asking the patient about the presence of risk factors, such as a family history of Alzheimer's disease and a history of head trauma, as well as asking about other pertinent clinical information, including a history of a psychiatric disorder, current or past use of substances, history of exposure to environmental toxins, and current use of over-the-counter medications (16). When the patient has mild or moderate impairments, a series of evaluations may be needed before the clinician can say with reasonable certainty that dementia is present.

For the most part, the physical examination is nonspecific. Focal neurological signs suggest previous strokes, mass lesions, or Parkinson's disease.

If the practitioner notes a history of decline, he or she should perform a screening test to further assess the patient's cognitive abilities. One of the easiest instruments to use is the Mini-Mental

State Exam (MMSE) (17). See Figure 4–1 for an example. The exam has a total score of 30 points, and it can be used to establish a baseline level of performance and to determine how a patient changes over time. A score between 19 and 23 indicates mild dementia, and a score of less than 18 indicates severe dementia (18). However, because performance on the exam is influenced by age, ethnicity, language, and visual or hearing impairment, scores—particularly those in the mild range—need to be interpreted with caution. The MMSE score cannot be used alone to diagnose dementia; it is to be used as data to support the history.

Neuropsychological testing is a standardized set of exams that measures various cognitive functions. It is not used routinely, but it has a number of indications, particularly in the assessment of patients with suspected early dementia who perform well on the MMSE or of patients in whom it is difficult to distinguish depression from dementia. These tests also provide useful information when decisions need to be made about the patient's safety (e.g., while driving) and competence (10).

Controversy exists about which laboratory tests to use to clarify the diagnosis. Members of the National Institute of Aging, the National Institute of Neurological and Communicative Disorders and Stroke, and the National Institute of Mental Health have recommended the tests listed in Table 4–2 (16).

If appropriate risk factors are present, the clinician should order a human immunodeficiency virus antibody test. The American Academy of Neurology has recommended that neuroimaging be performed at least once during the evaluation of any patient with suspected dementia (10).

Major depression can be confused with dementia. The symptoms of depression are similar in the elderly and in younger patients, but the elderly are more likely to complain of weight loss and decreased pleasure and are less likely to complain of guilt or feelings of worthlessness (19). The elderly may also emphasize somatic complaints instead of depressed mood. The depressive symptoms develop over several weeks, whereas the symptoms of dementia evolve over months to years.

Orientation

5 points ( ) What is the (year) (season) (date) (day) (month)?

5 points ( ) Which (country) (state) (town) (hospital) (floor) are we in/on?

Registration

3 points ( ) Name three objects, using 1 second to say each. Then ask the patient all three after you have said them. Give 1 point for each correct answer. Then repeat them until he or she learns all three. Count trials and record.

Attention and calculation

5 points ( ) Serial 7s. Give 1 point for each correct. Stop after five answers. Alternatively, ask patient to spell *world* backward.

Recall

3 points ( ) Ask for the three objects repeated in the Registration part of the exam. Give 1 point for each correct.

Language

9 points ( ) Name a pencil and a watch (2 points)

( ) Repeat the following: "No ifs, ands, or buts." (1 point)

( ) Follow a three-stage command:

"Take a paper in your right hand, fold it in half, and put it on the floor." (3 points)

Read and obey the following:

( ) Close your eyes (1 point)

( ) Write a sentence (1 point)

( ) Copy design (1 point)

_________Total score

FIGURE 4–1. **Mini-Mental State Exam.**
Source. Adapted from Folstein et al. 1975 (17).

TABLE 4–2. **Laboratory tests for the evaluation of dementia**
Complete blood count
Electrolyte panel
Metabolic panel
Thyroid function tests
B_{12} and folate levels
Syphilis serology
Urinalysis
Electrocardiogram
Chest X ray

Depressed patients may complain of memory problems, and cognitive changes may be noted on examination. These changes are referred to as *dementia of depression* or *pseudodementia.* These impairments are not as pervasive or as severe as those of Alzheimer's disease or other dementias, and with treatment, they resolve.

More common than the dementia of depression is the coexistence of major depression and Alzheimer's disease. Depression occurs in approximately 25% of patients with Alzheimer's disease, especially in patients in the early phases of dementia or in those who have concurrent medical problems or who abuse substances (18). A risk factor for developing depression during the course of Alzheimer's disease is a family history of depression (18). Treatment of the depression may improve mood and functioning, but cognitive impairment persists.

Delirium can also be confused with dementia. Delirium and dementia can occur simultaneously. The risk factors for delirium include dementia (20), severe illness, advanced age, and physical impairments (18). Delirium differs from dementia in that the onset of delirium is acute, it is seen mostly in hospitalized patients, the symptoms fluctuate throughout the day, and the course is brief. The symptoms include distractibility, disorientation, a change in the level of consciousness, and auditory or visual hallucinations (2).

Delirium suggests a significant, acute underlying process, such as pneumonia, congestive heart failure, or alcohol or sedative-hypnotic intoxication or withdrawal, but the most common cause is medications, even at therapeutic dosages (3). The medications most frequently implicated are anticholinergics, sedative-hypnotics, and narcotics (20). A common laboratory abnormality seen in delirious patients is hypoalbuminemia (20). If a patient with dementia suddenly becomes more confused, agitated, or lethargic or begins to hallucinate, the practitioner should be alerted to the presence of delirium and investigate for possible etiologies.

■ TREATMENT

Cognitive Symptoms

Except for vascular dementia, for which treatment is directed at preventing strokes, no preventive treatment exists for the irreversible dementias. However, some promising but preliminary developments have been made. One development is the use of antioxidant agents. One study showed that α-tocopherol (vitamin E) and selegiline, a monoamine oxidase inhibitor, may delay the progression of Alzheimer's disease (21). Another development is the discovery that estrogen stimulates the growth of neurons and improves cognition (22). More studies are needed before antioxidants or estrogen can be safely recommended for patients with early dementia.

Because of the link between acetylcholine and memory in Alzheimer's disease, researchers have studied several medications that increase acetylcholine in the central nervous system. The first such medication was tetrahydroaminoacridine (tacrine), a systemic acetylcholinesterase inhibitor. The response is dose dependent, and a dosage of at least 80 mg/day is necessary for therapeutic effects (23). Studies using tetrahydroaminoacridine showed modest improvement for brief periods in patients with mild to moderate dementia, but in studies involving longer trials, many patients stopped taking the medicine because of side effects, including hepatotoxicity, nausea, vomiting, and diarrhea. Because of the medication's hepatotoxicity, frequent monitoring of liver function is recommended.

Recently, another acetylcholinesterase inhibitor, donepezil (Aricept), was introduced for patients with mild to moderate dementia. Donepezil inhibits acetylcholine esterase only in the central nervous system. Its most frequent side effects are nausea, vomiting, diarrhea, and dizziness. It is not associated with hepatotoxicity (24). The recommended dosage is 5 mg/day. If the patient does not respond within 6 weeks, the dosage should be increased to 10 mg/day. The trial should be terminated if the patient has not responded within 3 months of initiation of therapy. If possible, the practitioner should consult a psychiatrist or neurologist before prescribing either of the acetylcholinesterase inhibitors.

Associated Symptoms

Behavioral and psychotic symptoms are frequently seen during the course of dementia. Before medications are considered as treatment for these symptoms, nonpharmacological means should be exhausted. For instance, because demented patients cannot interpret environmental stimuli quickly and may react aggressively, their lives should be routinized as much as possible, including scheduled meals, toileting, naps, and exercise. Their surroundings and caregivers should be as familiar and as consistent as possible. Well-lit rooms reduce *sundowning,* which is an exacerbation of disorientation that occurs in the evening hours. Hearing and visual impairments should be addressed, because patients with such impairments are apt to become paranoid (3). If wandering is a problem, the door locks should be changed. Stove burners can be fixed so that they are less easily manipulated. The patient should have no access to matches, cigarettes, or firearms (5).

Agitation, combativeness, delusions, and hallucinations are responsive to medications, whereas public disrobing, hoarding, repetitive questioning, screaming, and wandering are not (25, 26).

When prescribing medications, the practitioner should select a target symptom, initiate the lowest possible dosage, and then increase the dosage slowly. As the dementia progresses, the need for medication may change; the use of psychotropics should be reviewed every 6 months. Table 4–3 lists medications used to treat symptoms associated with dementia.

Neuroleptics are the treatment of choice for agitation, hallucinations, and delusions (26). No one neuroleptic is superior to another, and the choice should be based on side-effect profile. The lower-potency neuroleptics such as chlorpromazine have anticholinergic effects that may exacerbate impaired cognition. The higher-potency neuroleptics such as haloperidol (Haldol) may cause extrapyramidal side effects. If the patient remains agitated or psychotic after a 6- to 8-week trial of an adequate dosage of an antipsychotic, then the patient should be referred to a psychiatrist.

TABLE 4–3. **Medications used to treat symptoms associated with dementia**

Symptom	Medication	Daily dosage (mg)
Agitation	Chlorpromazine (Thorazine)	10–50
	Haloperidol (Haldol)	0.5–5
	Trazodone (Desyrel)	25–400
Hallucination, delusions	Chlorpromazine (Thorazine)	10–50
	Haloperidol (Haldol)	0.5–5
	Risperidone (Risperdal)	0.5–3
	Olanzapine (Zyprexa)	10
Major depression	Fluoxetine (Prozac)	10–20
	Sertraline (Zoloft)	25–150
	Paroxetine (Paxil)	10–20
	Venlafaxine (Effexor)	50–75
	Nefazodone (Serzone)	100–200
Sleep disturbance	Temazepam (Restoril)	15
	Zolpidem (Ambien)	5–10

New antipsychotics, such as risperidone (Risperdal) and olanzapine (Zyprexa), may cause fewer extrapyramidal symptoms and be better tolerated. These medications should not be used without the initial assistance of a psychiatrist.

Several alternatives to the antipsychotics are available for the treatment of agitation, including trazodone (Desyrel), buspirone (BuSpar), propranolol (Inderal), carbamazepine (Tegretol), and lithium carbonate. Trazodone can be used in divided daily doses as listed in Table 4–3, but the other medications listed should not be used without some guidance from a psychiatric colleague. The use of carbamazepine and lithium requires monitoring of blood levels and other parameters. Benzodiazepines can be used if anxiety is part of the agitation (26).

Because depression can further compromise quality of life in demented patients, pharmacological treatment is indicated and should be used empirically when the practitioner cannot separate symptoms of depression from those of dementia. As with the antipsychotics, the initial dosages of antidepressants should be low and increased gradually. The selective serotonin reuptake inhibitors (SSRIs) are easy to use and well tolerated. Commonly prescribed SSRIs include fluoxetine (Prozac), sertraline (Zoloft), and paroxetine (Paxil). Other recently released antidepressants are discussed in Chapter 1.

Changes in sleep architecture occur with aging and are exaggerated in Alzheimer's disease such that the patient experiences less deep sleep (3). Benzodiazepines can be used as hypnotics, but they may worsen cognition, cause paradoxical agitation, or produce dependence. They are best used for brief trials of 2–4 weeks. Other agents used to treat sleeplessness are trazodone and zolpidem.

It may be necessary for the clinician to consult a psychiatrist sometime during the course of treatment—for example, if the clinician suspects early dementia and seeks corroboration or more extensive evaluation, if he or she has difficulty separating symptoms of depression or delirium from those of dementia, or if he or she does not note improvement in a target symptom after an adequate trial of a medication. Psychiatric collaboration is also helpful in working with patients who exhibit cognitive problems but also have an extensive psychiatric history, for example, of schizophrenia or recurrent major depression.

Family involvement is crucial. Appointments should include time to talk to family members about what they have observed of the patient. Several helpful and easily available books have been written for families (e.g., *The 36-Hour Day* by Mace and Rabins [27]). Families should also be referred to the National Alzheimer's Association at (800) 272-3900 for information about support groups and referral to a local chapter.

Because dementia is a chronic disorder, patients and families should be educated about what to expect as the disease progresses and how to plan for the future. This education should include a discussion of advance directives, durable power of attorney, and institutionalization. Families may also ask about in-home nursing services and respite facilities (3). Because of the enormous stress associated with having a relative with dementia, family members may develop a major depression, and appropriate treatment or referrals should be initiated.

■ CONCLUSION

Most dementias are irreversible. As the dementia advances, behavioral, affective, or psychotic symptoms may develop. Some of these symptoms are amenable to pharmacotherapy, others to environmental changes. New agents are being developed to slow the progression of Alzheimer's disease. The dementias are devastating to patients and their families, and appropriate referrals need to be made.

■ REFERENCES

1. Katzman R: Alzheimer's disease. N Engl J Med 314:964–973, 1986
2. American Psychiatric Association: Diagnostic and Statistical Manual of Mental Disorders, 4th Edition. Washington, DC, American Psychiatric Association, 1994

3. Winograd CH, Jarvik LF: Physician management of the demented patient. J Am Geriatr Soc 34:295–308, 1986
4. Campion E: When a mind dies. N Engl J Med 334:791–792, 1996
5. Larson E, Lo B, Williams M: Evaluation and care of elderly patients with dementia. J Gen Intern Med 1:116–126, 1986
6. Butler RN, Finkel SI, Lewis MI, et al: Aging and mental health: diagnosis of dementia and depression. Geriatrics 47:49–57, 1992
7. Reisberg B: Dementia: a systemic approach to identifying reversible causes. Geriatrics 41:430–446, 1986
8. Doraiswamy PM, Steffens DC, Pitchumoni S, et al: Early recognition of Alzheimer's disease: what is consensual? what is controversial? what is practical? J Clin Psychiatry 59 (suppl 13):6–18, 1998
9. Fleming KC, Adams AC, Petersen RC: Dementia: diagnosis and evaluation. Mayo Clin Proc 70:1093–1107, 1995
10. Corey-Bloom J, Thal LJ, Galasko D, et al: Diagnosis and evaluation of dementia. Neurology 45:211–218, 1995
11. de la Monte SM, Ghanbari K, Frey WH, et al: Characterization of the AD7c-NTP cDNA expression in Alzheimer's disease and measurement of a 41-kD protein in cerebrospinal fluid. J Clin Invest 100: 3093–3104, 1997
12. Geldmacher DS, Whitehouse PJ: Evaluation of dementia. N Engl J Med 335:330–336, 1996
13. Mayeux R, Chun M: Acquired and hereditary dementias, in Merritt's Textbook of Neurology, 9th Edition. Edited by Rowland LP. Baltimore, MD, Williams & Wilkins, 1995, pp 677–685
14. Rossor M: The dementias, in Neurology in Clinical Practice, Vol 2: The Neurological Disorders. Edited by Bradley WG, Daroff RB, Fenichel GM, et al. Boston, MA, Butterworth- Heineman, 1989, pp 1407–1435
15. Charness ME, Simon RP, Greenberg DA: Ethanol and the nervous system. N Engl J Med 321:442–454, 1989
16. Consensus conference: differential diagnosis of dementing diseases. JAMA 258:3411–3416, 1987
17. Folstein MF, Folstein SE, McHugh PR: "Mini-mental state": a practical method for grading the cognitive state of patients for the clinician. J Psychiatr Res 12:189–198, 1975
18. Jones BN, Reifler BV: Depression co-existing with dementia: evaluation and treatment. Med Clin North Am 78:823–840, 1994
19. Blazer D: Depression in the elderly. N Engl J Med 320:164–166, 1989

20. Francis J: Delirium in older patients. J Am Geriatr Soc 40:829–839, 1992
21. Sano M, Ernest C, Thomas RG, et al: A controlled trial of selegiline, alpha-tocopherol, or both as treatment for Alzheimer's disease. N Engl J Med 336:1216–1222, 1997
22. Wickelgren I: Estrogen stakes claim to cognition. Science 276:675–678, 1997
23. Schneider LS, Tariot P: Emerging drugs for Alzheimer's disease: mechanism of action and prospects for cognitive enhancing medications. Med Clin North Am 78:911–934, 1994
24. Rogers SL, Friedhoff LT: The efficacy and safety of donepezil in patients with Alzheimer's disease: results of a US multicentre, randomized, double-blind, placebo-controlled trial. The Donepezil Study Group. Dementia 7:293–303, 1996
25. Johnson J, Sims R, Gottlieb G: Differential diagnosis of dementia, delirium, and depression. Drugs Aging 5:431–445, 1994
26. Sky AJ, Grossberg G: The use of psychotropic medication in the management of problem behaviors in the patient with Alzheimer's disease. Med Clin North Am 78:811–822, 1994
27. Mace NL, Robins PV: The 36-Hour Day, Revised Edition. Baltimore, MD, Johns Hopkins University Press, 1991

5

SOMATOFORM AND RELATED DISORDERS

Sarah Gelbach DeMichele, M.D.
James L. Stinnett, M.D.

Patients may exhibit physical symptoms that the practitioner cannot explain using his or her knowledge of disease processes. These patients are often called difficult, hysterical, or psychosomatic (1). Psychological problems, though not overtly stated, are often an issue for such patients. Between 25% and 75% of patient complaints to their primary care practitioners represent somatic manifestations of psychological distress (2).

Somatization is the process by which the patient unconsciously manifests physical symptoms or signs to satisfy a psychological need. In the primary care setting, psychiatric illnesses such as depression, anxiety, panic, schizophrenia, and the personality disorders may manifest themselves as somatic symptoms (3). Eighty percent of depressed or anxious patients experience only somatic symptoms (4). Over time, the recognizable psychiatric symptoms of these disorders predominate over the somatic symptoms. Early awareness of somatization as a manifestation of these disorders is vital to proper diagnosis and effective treatment. Once the underlying disorder is treated, the somatic symptoms may resolve (5).

The somatoform disorders—somatization disorder, conversion disorder, hypochondriasis, body dysmorphic disorder, and pain disorder—have somatization as a primary component. In this chapter, we describe the specific characteristics and manifestations of each of these disorders. We also discuss factitious disorder, malingering, and delusional disorder of the somatic type. Table 5–1 summarizes the somatoform and related disorders (6).

Patients who have physical complaints that cannot be attributed easily to a specific disease put great demands on the health care system. These patients are often overstudied in that physicians and patients alike pursue extensive diagnostic workups. One study reported a 6-fold increase in hospital costs and a 14-fold increase in physician charges for patients diagnosed as having a somatoform disorder (7). This study also found an absence of life-threatening

TABLE 5–1. **Somatoform and related disorders**

Disorder	Characteristics
Somatization disorder	Many physical complaints, particularly of pain and of gastrointestinal, neurological, and sexual symptoms
Conversion disorder	Symptoms involve motor or sensory function; psychological conflicts or stressors precede the onset of symptoms
Hypochondriasis	Preoccupation (but not a delusion) that one has a serious illness; preoccupation persists despite thorough evaluation and reassurance
Body dysmorphic disorder	Preoccupation (but not a delusion) with an imagined or exaggerated physical deformity
Pain disorder	Pain symptoms produce significant impairment; psychological factors are involved in onset and perpetuation of pain symptoms
Factitious disorder	Physical or mental symptoms are feigned to assume the sick role
Malingering	Physical or mental symptoms are feigned to avoid responsibilities, for financial gain, or for medications
Delusional disorder of the somatic type	Delusions that one has a general medical condition or physical defect

pathology that could justify the increased health care expenditures (7). The physician, frustrated that the patient's symptoms have no explanation, may order studies that are increasingly sophisticated, expensive, and risky. The patient, also unsatisfied with the diagnostic results, can increase pressure on the physician to make a diagnosis and often "doctor shops" in search of an answer. This process, which focuses only on the patient's symptoms and not on psychological factors, places the patient at greater risk for iatrogenic complications. It also reinforces the very symptoms the physician and the patient were hoping to eliminate.

People who have these disorders can exhaust clinicians because they make frequent appointments, phone calls, emergency room visits, and require repeated hospitalizations. Their need for reassurance and attention can be overwhelming to practitioners. Both practitioners and patients can feel angry, frustrated, tense, and hopeless. The combination of the "demanding dependency and unresponsiveness to treatment" (8, p. 413) is difficult to comprehend, because it contradicts the expectation of recovery.

■ SPECIFIC SOMATOFORM DISORDERS

Patients with somatoform disorders exhibit physical symptoms unconsciously, as a socially, culturally, or personally acceptable expression of their internal psychological distress. The symptoms may be significant enough to cause functional impairment and disability. Note that these patients are a heterogeneous group and that diagnostic overlap exists between these disorders. Comorbidity exists between the somatoform disorders and other psychiatric disorders, such as mood and anxiety disorders. Also, documented medical illnesses may be present in addition to the unexplained somatic symptoms.

Somatization Disorder

Somatization disorder is more common in females, begins by age 30, and is characterized not only by a constellation of many symptoms representing many organ systems but also by its chronicity. Estimates indicate that somatization disorder may be present in 5%–10% of patients seen in primary care settings (9). By DSM-IV criteria, the patient must have experienced each of the following: four pain symptoms, two gastrointestinal symptoms, one sexual symptom, and one neurological symptom (6). Either these symptoms are inexplicable medically or the patient experiences distress out of proportion to the documented pathophysiology. Common symptoms include chest pain, palpitations, abdominal bloating, depressed feelings, dizziness, weakness, and difficulty breathing (7). Often the patient tells dramatic and emotional stories characterized by multiple physician contacts, medications, diagnostic tests, and surgeries. Somatic complaints are sustained over time, although the specific symptom complex and the intensity of the symptoms may vary. The patient's perception of disability is striking.

Conversion Disorder

Conversion disorder can occur at any age, is episodic, and has a female predominance, but in contrast to somatization disorder, it is more episodic in nature (9). Conversion disorder is defined as the presence of one or more neurological symptoms that cannot be explained by conventional testing and the identification of precipitating psychological factors. Four subtypes exist: motor, sensory, seizure, and mixed symptomatology (6). Often the symptom has a symbolic meaning; for example, a patient may develop so-called hysterical blindness after witnessing a tragic event. A significant number of patients meeting the criteria for conversion disorder are eventually given a neurological or medical diagnosis (10). For instance, one-third of patients diagnosed as having pseudoseizures also have epilepsy (9). Vigilance for neurological and medical pathology must be maintained. Between 90% and 100% of patients experience symptom resolution within 1 month, although 25% may have a recurrence (9).

Hypochondriasis

Hypochondriasis, in contrast to the other somatoform disorders, has an equal incidence in males and females (6). The distinguishing feature of hypochondriasis is the fear of disease rather than a focus on specific symptoms. These patients exhibit *somatosensory amplification,* which has three components: 1) hypervigilance to normal and abnormal bodily sensations; 2) a focus on weak, infrequent sensations; and 3) a tendency to attribute abnormal pathological meaning to the sensations (4).

Patients with hypochondriasis range from the transient to the persistent worrier (11). The persistent hypochondriac experiences significant medical and psychiatric morbidity and impairment but does not use significantly more mental health resources (12). These patients continuously seek reassurance from their physicians that they are not ill, although reassurance fails to relieve their preoccupations. Frequent outpatient visits, phone calls, and doctor shopping is the rule rather than the exception. Although hypochondriasis diminishes the patient's functional ability and causes great anxiety, by definition the preoccupation stops short of becoming delusional. Exaggerated beliefs of illness diminish over time in 50% of patients (12).

Body Dysmorphic Disorder

Body dysmorphic disorder is defined as a person's preoccupation with an imagined physical defect (6). It often begins in late adolescence and affects females predominately. Although gradual in onset, the preoccupation goes beyond mere dissatisfaction. The patient's occupational and social functioning become impaired significantly, as he or she imagines the reactions of others to the perceived deformity and then avoids interpersonal interactions (6). Up to one-third of these patients may be housebound (9). The most common concern is facial deformity, and these patients may account for 2% of those presenting to plastic surgeons (13). This disorder is distinct from anorexia nervosa and transsexualism, even though these disorders also include a component of dissatisfaction with perceived defects or deformities (6). Pharmacotherapy with serotonergic agents such as clomipramine (Anafranil) and fluoxetine (Prozac) is effective in patients with body dysmorphic disorder, reducing symptoms in 50% of patients (9).

Pain Disorder

Pain disorder is characterized by one or more pain symptoms that have been significant enough for the patient to seek medical care and that cause distress and functional impairment. Identifiable psychological factors are deemed to be important in the initiation and maintenance of the symptoms. The disorder is further classified into subtypes that distinguish between pain associated with a general medical condition that partially explains the degree of impairment and pain reported in patients without an associated medical diagnosis (6). The pain these patients report is unrelenting and often shows little improvement, even temporarily with analgesia. These patients doctor shop, often take multiple medications, and may desire surgical intervention. A substantial proportion of them have concomitant depressive disorders.

■ FACTITIOUS DISORDERS

Patients with factitious disorders deliberately report, feign, or produce symptoms or signs of medical illnesses. Patients who have somatoform disorders or factitious disorders unconsciously want to be in a relationship with a physician or health care professional. However, patients with somatoform disorders do not feign symptoms; to them, the symptoms develop spontaneously. Patients with factitious disorders plan ways in which to have medical problems, although they are unable to explain their actions.

Factitious disorders are seen in up to 5% of patient encounters (14). These patients are predominately female and often have health care knowledge or a background in health care (15). They are willing to accept invasive, uncomfortable procedures and undergo surgical intervention without protest (15).

The presenting symptoms may be psychological or physical, subjective or objective. Examples include a patient who surreptitiously takes diuretics to produce hypokalemia, a patient who complains of flank pain and who then puts blood in a urine specimen to feign nephrolithiasis, a patient who pricks him- or herself repeatedly to produce nonhealing skin ulcers, or a patient who feigns auditory hallucinations. The primary motivation is the opportunity to take on the sick role and benefit from the attention, mastery, caring, and dependency that the role affords these patients (15). On the surface, these patients enact their medical dramas primarily to assume and then legitimize their role as patients who can then be admitted to hospitals and be treated with invasive diagnostic and therapeutic procedures. However, they engage in these repetitive dramas for exceedingly complex and unconscious reasons. Although the symptoms themselves are feigned intentionally, the behavior has an involuntary and compulsive quality.

Factitious disorders can be incapacitating, and the prognosis is poor, although less so when the disorders occur with other more readily treatable psychiatric disorders such as depression (15). Poor prognostic indicators are antisocial personality traits and bizarre behavior (15). Early recognition of these disorders is essential for treatment, which consists of managing the symptoms, without the expectation of a cure, and limiting the number of invasive, risky diagnostic procedures. These patients frustrate and infuriate health care providers, because they are often thought to be wasting the provider's time and other health care resources. Factitious disorders, although not a diagnosis of exclusion, must be differentiated from physical disease, somatoform disorders, personality disorders, schizophrenia, and malingering.

Munchausen syndrome is a striking variant of the factitious disorders, characterized by a complex, intriguing, and plausible story; extensive traveling to pursue medical workups; and pathological lying. Patients with this syndrome have traits of borderline and antisocial personality disorders and engage in drug-seeking behavior (15).

■ MALINGERING

Malingering is not a type of factitious disorder, although these patients also feign illnesses. The main motivation for malingerers is not the establishment of a relationship with a practitioner or to be in the hospital but to achieve an external gain, such as financial compensation, access to controlled substances, or avoidance of legal, family, or work-related responsibilities. These patients are capable of explaining their behavior, but they choose not to do so. Practitioners are often infuriated with these patients because of their duplicity.

■ DELUSIONAL DISORDER

Delusional disorder of the somatic type can also be seen in primary care practices. Patients with somatic delusions exhibit firmly held, nonbizarre ideas regarding medical illnesses, such as infestation, halitosis, and emission of bodily odors. The symptoms are distressing and may cause patients to limit their social interactions. The delusions, although intense, are well circumscribed. Patients with delusions of parasitosis are predominantly middle-aged women (16), whereas those with delusions of halitosis are predominately men (17). Delusions of infestation can be associated with amphetamine, methylphenidate (Ritalin), and cocaine abuse (17).

Delusional disorder of the somatic type must be differentiated from other psychiatric, medical, and neurological disorders. Neuroleptics are the treatment of choice, although patients may be reluctant to take them. Pimozide (Orap) is the neuroleptic of choice for somatic delusions; 82% of patients report a remission of symptoms, often within 2 weeks (18).

■ MANAGEMENT OF THE DOCTOR-PATIENT RELATIONSHIP IN PATIENTS WITH SOMATOFORM AND RELATED DISORDERS

Patients who have unexplained medical symptoms are often difficult to work with because of the psychological and social gains they derive by being ill. Somatic presentations decrease the likelihood that an associated primary psychiatric disorder will be diagnosed (3). Treatment of somatic disorders in the primary care setting requires that the practitioner consider a comprehensive biopsychosocial model of illness. Identifying the symptom as a somatic manifestation of psychological distress is the first step in a long and difficult therapeutic process. As mentioned earlier in this chapter, practitioners are often frustrated by these patients, but understanding that psychologically determined distress can interfere with a patient's life as much as distress from a physical process may help to diminish some of these negative reactions. Goals of treatment are to diminish the patient's distress, to increase his or her functional ability, to decrease symptoms, and to reduce his or her inappropriate use of medical care (19).

The management of these challenging patients includes several components (see Table 5–2). The suggestions listed in Chapter 7 also apply.

1. The key to establishing a healthy therapeutic alliance with these patients is to schedule regular, frequent appointments that are independent of symptom exacerbation. The practitioner thus conveys that he or she is taking the patient seriously and that changing or amplifying symptoms is unnecessary to get an appointment.
2. Practitioners must realize that these patients are seeking care, not a cure. The goal of the therapeutic relationship should not and cannot be to completely eliminate the symptom or the underlying disorder but rather should be to improve the patient's functional status and reduce long-term morbidity. Practitioners should emphasize that the symptoms may be present to some degree in the future and that the therapeutic goal is to make the symptoms bearable (20). The patient may initially react negatively to this approach and may be frustrated by the lack of immediate action. Telling the patient that if there were a "quick fix" it would have been done already may help him or her accept a more chronic course of treatment (20).

TABLE 5–2. **Treatment recommendations for patients with somatoform and related disorders**
Schedule regular, frequent appointments even if the patient feels well
Make maintenance of care, not cure, the goal of treatment
Evaluate the patient for other psychiatric disorders—for example, major depression
Make follow-up visits brief and structured
Use medication if indicated
Emphasize improving functional abilities
Introduce the idea of stressors by asking about the patient's daily life
Use psychiatric consultation judiciously
Facilitate frequent communication between primary care practitioner and psychiatrist
Use appropriate limit setting when malingering is suspected

3. Physicians should listen to the patient's somatic complaints but should also be alert for comorbid psychopathology, namely depression and anxiety, and for signs or symptoms of true organic pathology. Appropriate treatment or consultations should be undertaken as indicated. Direct confrontation or immediate attribution of psychological explanations is rarely useful (20). Over time, with the practitioner's attention to the biological, psychological, and social aspects of the patient's health, many patients will be amenable to some degree of psychosocial explanation for their physical symptoms.
4. Follow-up visits should be brief and structured. The practitioner should briefly review the patient's symptoms and should not expect the symptoms to diminish. In the initial follow-up stages, the symptoms may even increase in severity, which will test the practitioner's interest in continuing to care for the patient. Diagnostic tests should be administered when indicated.
5. Medication management of these patients can be complicated. Appropriate medication for defined psychiatric conditions such as anxiety and depression is clearly indicated. The use of such medications may require psychiatric referral. Other

medication choices should be made with the specific goals of diminishing symptoms to improve functional ability. Medication trials should be time limited. Narcotics should be avoided because of abuse potential (20). Sedative-hypnotics, if necessary, should be used for brief periods only.

6. The focus should be on improving the patient's functional ability. Treatment can be developed that encourages the patient to improve his or her daily function in ways that are meaningful to the individual—for example, making the bed 4 days a week or walking one block each day.
7. An exploration of the interplay between the psychosocial stressors and the physical symptoms the patient experiences can begin only in the context of a trusting therapeutic relationship. It may be helpful to introduce the topic by discussing the psychological effect of the reported symptoms. For instance, the practitioner can ask the patient how the symptoms interfere with family life or work. This approach does not directly challenge the patient's assumptions that the symptoms are physical, and it may increase the patient's comfort and familiarity with the language of emotional expressions rather than somatic ones.
8. Discussion with the patient of the utility of a psychiatric consultation may be indicated. Often, patients will feel threatened, believing that the physician has finally tired of them and is dumping them on a colleague. The primary care practitioner must reinforce that he or she will continue to follow the patient closely and that the psychiatrist is a consultant only.
9. Successful collaboration between primary care practitioners and psychiatrists depends on frequent communication and, if indicated, joint sessions with the patient. This approach reinforces for the patient that psychiatric and medical approaches are necessary for treatment.
10. If the practitioner suspects that a patient is malingering, confrontation rarely helps the patient. Such a step usually elicits from the patient denial, evasion, or an angry outburst. Instead, the practitioner should deny requests that he or she feels are

unreasonable, such as requests for controlled substances, unnecessary tests, or letters excusing the patient from responsibilities.

CONCLUSION

Patients who somatize or feign symptoms unconsciously seek a caring relationship with a health care provider. It is often frustrating to work with these patients, but by integrating a psychological understanding of these patients with somatic interventions, primary care practitioners can make caring for these patients more rewarding.

REFERENCES

1. Kahn SR, Crone K, Spitfire RL, et al: The difficult patient: prevalence, psychopathology and functional impairment. J Gen Intern Med 11:1–8, 1996
2. Katon W, Ries RK, Kleinman A: The prevalence of somatization in primary care. Compr Psychiatry 25:208–215, 1984
3. Kirmayer LJ, Robbins JM, Dworkind M, et al: Somatization and the recognition of depression and anxiety in primary care. Am J Psychiatry 150:734–741, 1993
4. Barsky AJ: Amplification, somatization and the somatoform disorders. Psychosomatics 33:28–34, 1992
5. Stinnett JL: The functional somatic symptom. Psychiatr Clin North Am 10:19–33, 1987
6. American Psychiatric Association: Diagnostic and Statistical Manual of Mental Disorders, 4th Edition. Washington, DC, American Psychiatric Association, 1994
7. Smith GR, Monson RA, Ray D: Patients with multiple unexplained symptoms: their characteristics, functional health, and health care utilization. Arch Intern Med 146:69–72, 1986
8. Barsky AJ, Wyshak G, Latham KS, et al: Hypochondriacal patients, their physicians and their medical care. J Gen Intern Med 6:413–419, 1991
9. Kaplan HI, Sadock BJ, Grebb JA: Somatoform disorders, in Synopsis of Psychiatry, 7th Edition. Baltimore, MD, Williams & Wilkins, 1994, pp 617–637
10. Lazare A: Conversion symptoms. N Engl J Med 305:745–748, 1981

11. Kellner R: Diagnosis and treatment of hypochondriacal syndromes. Psychosomatics 33:278–289, 1992
12. Robbins JM, Kirmayer LJ: Transient and persistent hypochondriacal worry in primary care. Psychol Med 26:575–589, 1996
13. Hollander E, Neville D, Frenkel M, et al: Body dysmorphic disorder: diagnostic issues and related disorders. Psychosomatics 33:156–165, 1992
14. Wallach J: Laboratory diagnosis of factitious disorders. Arch Intern Med 154:1690–1696, 1994
15. Folks DG: Munchausen's syndrome and other factitious disorders. Neurol Clin 13:267–278, 1995
16. Koo J, Gambla C: Delusions of parasitosis and other forms of monosymptomatic hypochondriacal psychosis: general discussion and case illustrations. Dermatol Clin 14:429–438, 1996
17. Baker PB, Cook BL, Winoker G: Delusional infestation: the interface of delusions and hallucinations. Psychiatr Clin North Am 18:345–361, 1995
18. Munro A: Monosymptomatic hypochondriacal psychosis. Br J Psychiatry 153 (suppl 2):37–40, 1988
19. Mayou R: Somatization. Psychother Psychosom 59:69–83, 1993
20. Kaplan C, Lipkin M, Gordon GH: Somatization in primary care: patients with unexplained and vexing medical complaints. J Gen Intern Med 3:177–190, 1988

6

PSYCHOTIC DISORDERS

Stephan C. Mann, M.D.
Michael F. Gliatto, M.D.
E. Cabrina Campbell, M.D.
Robert A. Greenstein, M.D.

Psychosis is a broad term indicating a gross impairment in reality testing. Signs and symptoms include perceptual disturbances (i.e., hallucinations), delusions, disordered thought processes, and bizarre behavior. Psychosis is a feature of various psychiatric disorders (most notably schizophrenia) and a wide range of medical conditions and substance-induced disorders. In this chapter, we focus on the differentiation and management of psychosis associated with these diverse conditions.

■ GENERAL CHARACTERISTICS

Delusions

A delusion is a false belief based on incorrect inferences about external reality that is firmly maintained by the patient despite clear evidence to the contrary. Delusional beliefs are not attributable to the patient's social, cultural, or religious background. Patients may believe that they are being spied on or harmed in some way (persecutory delusions), that they have special powers or talents (grandiose delusions), or that some malignant process is occurring in their bodies (somatic delusions). Delusions of reference involve beliefs that remarks, statements, or items heard on television, on the radio, or in the street refer to or contain special messages for the patient. Certain bizarre delusions that indicate a loss of control over mind or body are particularly common in schizophrenia—for example, delusions of thoughts being inserted into or withdrawn from a patient's mind, delusions of thoughts being broadcast, and delusions of control by an outside force.

Hallucinations

Hallucinations are sensory perceptions that occur in the absence of external stimuli. They differ from illusions, which are misperceptions of real sensory stimuli. Hallucinations may be auditory, visual, tactile, gustatory, or olfactory. Auditory hallucinations are the type most frequently experienced in schizophrenia; the patient may describe buzzing, ringing, music, or, more typically, voices. Visual and other types of hallucinations in the absence of auditory hallucinations often suggest the involvement of a medical condition or substance use in the etiology of the psychosis.

Disordered Thought Processes

Thought disorders become apparent to the practitioner when he or she listens to the patient speak and respond to questions. In *circumstantiality,* questions are answered eventually, but the patient's response is excessively wordy and includes irrelevant detail. In *tangentiality,* the question is never answered because the patient continually strays from the intended point. However, in both circumstantiality and tangentiality, the patient's sentences are linked coherently. In *loosening of associations,* the patient's ideas shift from one subject to another in an unrelated way and his or her speech becomes increasingly incomprehensible. In its most severe form, loosening of associations may progress to incoherence. *Poverty of thought* involves speech that is brief and without detail. *Blocking* is observed when patients suddenly stop speaking and cannot recall what they were discussing prior to the pause. in *flight of ideas,* a nearly continuous flow of accelerated speech produces constant shifting from one idea to another, usually based on understandable associations, distracting stimuli, or play on words. *Neologisms* are words that are invented and have meaning only for the patient.

Disorganized Behavior

Psychotic patients may exhibit a variety of bizarre behaviors. They may act silly, agitated, or withdrawn, and they may appear disheveled or be oddly dressed. They may engage in inappropriately sexual or intrusive behavior (e.g., speaking directly into the interviewer's face). They may exhibit catatonia, which involves a complex of motor abnormalities, including immobility, excessive activity, voluntary assumption of bizarre postures, negativism, or mutism.

Positive and Negative Symptoms

Positive symptoms, such as delusions and hallucinations, reflect an excess or distortion of normal mental functions. In contrast, negative symptoms reflect a diminution or loss of normal mental functions. Negative symptoms include lack of spontaneity, blunted affect, lack of motivation, lack of social contacts, and inability to be persistent at work or school. Negative symptoms may be difficult to distinguish from depression and from some of the extrapyramidal side effects of antipsychotic medications.

■ PSYCHOSIS ASSOCIATED WITH A MEDICAL CONDITION OR SUBSTANCE USE

Virtually any cerebral, systemic, or substance-induced process that affects brain functioning can produce psychotic symptoms. In such cases, the diagnosis of psychotic disorder due to a general medical condition or of substance-induced psychotic disorder is made. (The term *substance* here refers to a drug of abuse, a medication, or a toxin.) We discuss some of these conditions in the sections that follow.

General Medical Conditions

Patients with psychotic disorder due to a general medical condition often exhibit features that are atypical for a primary psychiatric disorder (e.g., schizophrenia) such as older age at onset, lack of family history of a primary psychotic disorder, or visual or olfactory hallucinations. The etiologic role of a general medical condition in causing a psychotic disorder is supported by a temporal relationship between the onset, exacerbation, or remission of the general medical condition and that of the psychotic disorder. Psychotic disorders associated with a general medical condition often improve following treatment of the underlying disorder; however, this is not always the case. For example, psychosis due to hypothyroidism or infectious disease may not improve because of irreversible tissue damage (1). Table 6–1 summarizes selected causes of psychotic disorder due to a general medical condition. Neurological and endocrinological disorders are implicated frequently.

Neurological disorders. Much attention has been directed to chronic psychotic states developing between seizures in patients with complex partial seizures, most of which have a temporal lobe focus. These states emerge a mean of 14 years after the onset of seizures and are schizophrenia-like, but they involve preservation of appropriate affect and are not associated with the clinical deterioration of schizophrenia (2).

Basal ganglia diseases have a significant association with psychosis. Prevalence rates for delusions and psychosis are greater than 50% in Huntington's disease and idiopathic basal ganglia calcification and less than 25% in postencephalitic Parkinson's disease (3). Psychosis in idiopathic Parkinson's disease appears primarily as a result of depression associated with that disorder or as a result of antiparkinsonian drug treatment. New-onset psychosis may be the earliest manifestation of Wilson's disease.

Various acute and chronic infectious processes involving the central nervous system may cause psychotic symptoms. Viral encephalitis can manifest itself initially as an acute psychosis with

TABLE 6–1. **Selected causes of psychotic disorder due to a general medical condition**

Neurological disorders	**Endocrinological disorders**
Brain neoplasms	Adrenocortical insufficiency
Cerebrovascular disorders	Cushing's disease
Complex partial seizures	Hypo-/hyperparathyroidism
Deafness	Hypo-/hyperthyroidism
Head trauma	Panhypopituitarism
Huntington's disease	**Metabolic disorders**
Idiopathic basal ganglia calcification (Fahr's disease)	Acute intermittent porphyria
Infections (e.g., viral encephalitis, AIDS, neurosyphilis, Creutzfeldt-Jakob disease)	Electrolyte abnormalities (e.g., sodium, potassium, phosphate, calcium, magnesium)
Migraine	Hepatic encephalopathy
Normal-pressure hydrocephalus	Hypoxia
Parkinson's disease (idiopathic and postencephalitic)	Renal failure
Spinocerebellar degeneration	**Nutritional disorders**
Wilson's disease (hepatolenticular degeneration)	Folate deficiency
Autoimmune disorders	Malnutrition
Systemic lupus erythematosus	Niacin deficiency (pellagra)
	Thiamine deficiency (Wernicke-Korsakoff syndrome)
	Vitamin B_{12} deficiency

Note. AIDS = acquired immunodeficiency syndrome.

only subtle or minimal neurological findings. In some cases an acute psychosis has been the sole initial sign of infection with the human immunodeficiency virus (HIV) (4).

Endocrinological disorders. Psychosis may accompany hypothyroidism and at times may be the presenting complaint. Psychotic symptoms may also be seen in hyperthyroidism, particularly in severe cases or during thyroid storm (5). Psychosis has also been noted in disorders of the adrenals and parathyroid glands.

Substance-Induced Psychotic Disorders

Table 6–2 lists selected medications, toxins, and drugs of abuse associated with substance-induced psychotic disorder. The diagnosis of substance-induced psychotic disorder is not made if the patient is delirious. Substance-induced psychotic disorders arise in association with intoxication or withdrawal states. Individuals most at risk for developing psychotic disorders secondary to medications include the elderly, the medically ill, and those taking multiple medications (6). Many commonly used medications (both prescription and over-the-counter) are capable of producing psychotic symptoms. The emergence of psychosis may be related to the dosage or may be idiosyncratic (7). In addition, toxins such as pesticides containing anticholinesterase or organophosphates; nerve gas; carbon dioxide; carbon monoxide; and volatile substances such as fuel or paint can cause psychosis, as can intoxication with heavy metals such as mercury or manganese.

Substance-induced psychotic disorders are most commonly the result of intoxication or withdrawal involving drugs of abuse. Although generally associated with heavy drug use, these disorders may develop at low dosages in vulnerable individuals (8). In some instances, individuals vulnerable to developing psychotic symptoms after substance use also have underlying risk factors for psychiatric disorders such as schizophrenia (9). A complicating factor with substance-induced psychotic disorders is that many patients with psychiatric disorders abuse substances. As such, it is difficult to determine whether psychotic symptoms are induced by substances, a psychiatric disorder, or both.

■ PSYCHOSIS ASSOCIATED WITH A PSYCHIATRIC DISORDER

Psychiatric conditions that involve psychotic symptoms include schizophrenia and related conditions such as schizophreniform disorder, brief psychotic disorder, delusional disorder, and schizoaffective disorder. In addition, mood disorders (bipolar disorder

TABLE 6–2. **Selected causes of substance-induced psychotic disorder**

Category	Substance	Examples (where applicable)
Medications	Analgesics	Meperidine, pentazocine, salicylates (especially high dosages or in elderly patients), nonsteroidal anti-inflammatory drugs
	Anticholinergics	Antihistamines, antiparkinsonian anticholinergics, antipsychotics (especially thioridazine), antispasmodics, atropine eyedrops, tricyclic and tetracyclic antidepressants
	Antibiotics	Acyclovir, amphotericin B, cephalosporins, ciprofloxacin, metronidazole, penicillin G procaine
	Anticonvulsants	Carbamazepine, ethosuximide, phenobarbital, phenytoin, primidone, valproic acid; primarily in overdosages
	Antihypertensive and cardiovascular medications	Captopril, clonidine, digitalis, disopyramide, lidocaine, methyldopa, procainamide, propranolol, quinidine, reserpine, tocainide
	Antimalarials	Chloroquine, quinacrine
	Antineoplastics	Asparaginase, cyclosporine, 5-fluorouracil, procarbazine, vincristine
	Antiparkinsonian dopamine agonists	Amantadine, bromocriptine, L-dopa
	Antipsychotics	High-potency agents
	Antituberculous medications	Cycloserine, isoniazid, rifampin
	Baclofen	
	Cimetidine	

(continued)

TABLE 6–2. **Selected causes of substance-induced psychotic disorder *(continued)***

Category	Substance	Examples (where applicable)
Medications *(continued)*	Disulfiram	
	Glucocorticoids	
	Adrenocorticotropic hormone	
	Podophyllin (oral and cutaneous)	
	Thyroxine	
	Over-the-counter medications	Aminophylline, ephedrine, phenylpropanolamine, pseudoephedrine
Toxins	Anticholinesterase	
	Bromide	
	Carbon dioxide	
	Carbon monoxide	
	Heavy metals	Arsenic, bismuth, magnesium, manganese, mercury, thallium
	Nerve gas	
	Organophosphate insecticides	
	Volatile substances	Fuel, paint
Drugs of abuse	Alcohol (withdrawal)	
	Amphetamines	
	Anabolic steroids	
	Cannabis	

Cocaine	
Hallucinogens	LSD, mescaline
Inhalants	
Phencyclidine	
Sedative-hypnotics (withdrawal)	

and major depression) not uncommonly present with psychotic symptoms. Patients with personality disorders—especially borderline, narcissistic, histrionic, schizotypal, schizoid, or paranoid personality disorders—may experience transient psychotic symptoms when under stress (10). Furthermore, posttraumatic stress disorder and certain dissociative disorders may involve psychotic symptoms. Occasionally patients may feign psychosis to fulfill a need to assume the sick role (i.e., factitious disorder with psychological symptoms) or because of obvious external incentives (i.e., malingering).

Schizophrenia

Schizophrenia is the prototypical psychotic disorder. It has no single diagnostic sign or symptom. According to DSM-IV, schizophrenia is a disturbance that has persisted for at least 6 months and has included at least 1 month of at least two of the following symptoms: delusions, hallucinations, disorganized speech, grossly disorganized or catatonic behavior, or negative symptoms (11). In addition, the patient's social or occupational functioning must have declined to a level significantly lower than that prior to the onset of the disorder. Table 6–3 summarizes DSM-IV criteria for schizophrenia.

Schizophrenia affects approximately 1% of the population, with a male-to-female ratio close to 1:1 (12). Schizophrenia typically manifests itself between the teenage years and young adulthood and leads to severe and usually long-lasting impairment in most patients. Schizophrenia usually begins with a prodromal phase involving the insidious onset of social withdrawal, deterioration in grooming, loss of interest in school or work, and mild positive symptoms. An active phase of florid psychotic symptoms follows, marking the disturbance as schizophrenia and frequently bringing the patient to medical attention for the first time. The active phase resolves into a residual phase that is similar to the prodromal phase. Negative symptoms are common in the prodromal and residual phases. The residual phase may be followed by a re-

TABLE 6–3. Abbreviated DSM-IV criteria for schizophrenia

A. Characteristic (active phase) symptoms (at least two present for a significant portion of time during a 1-month period):

   (1) Delusions
   (2) Hallucinations
   (3) Disorganized speech (frequent derailment or incoherence)
   (4) Grossly disorganized or catatonic behavior
   (5) Negative symptoms (affective flattening, alogia, or avolition)

B. Impairment in social or occupational functioning

C. Duration of illness of at least 6 months, including at least 1 month of active phase symptoms

D. Schizoaffective disorder and mood disorder with psychotic features have been ruled out

E. Symptoms are not due to the direct physiologic effects of a substance or a general medical condition

Source. Adapted from American Psychiatric Association 1994 (11).

turn of active-phase symptoms (called an *acute exacerbation*). Many patients relapse and require rehospitalization.

Schizophrenia has a number of subtypes. The major feature of the paranoid type is prominent delusions or auditory hallucinations in the context of relative preservation of cognitive functioning and affect. This type has a better prognosis, and patients are more likely to be married and employed. The disorganized type has a very poor prognosis. These patients may appear silly, childlike, bizarre, and unkempt and are frequently unable to perform the basic activities of daily living. The catatonic type involves a clinical picture dominated by catatonic motor signs. In the undifferentiated type, no one of the above clinical presentations predominates.

Other Disorders

Other psychiatric disorders can be confused with schizophrenia. The differences between them can be subtle, but making the distinction is important because of disparate prognoses and approaches to treatment. When one of these disorders is suspected, it is best to refer the patient to a psychiatrist who can clarify the diagnosis and recommend the initial treatment plan.

Schizophreniform disorder. Schizophreniform disorder is identical to schizophrenia except that the symptoms have been present for only 1–6 months. In addition, impaired social or occupational functioning is not required for the practitioner to make the diagnosis. At least 25% of patients recover fully from an episode of schizophreniform disorder, although many relapse (11).

Brief psychotic disorder. Brief psychotic disorder involves the sudden onset of psychotic symptoms, frequently in response to a marked stressor. The symptoms are present from 1 day to 1 month and then remit completely. An example is postpartum psychosis, which occurs within 4 weeks of delivery. Patients with severe personality disorders are at risk for developing brief psychotic disorder.

Delusional disorder. Delusional disorder involves delusions that are not bizarre, such as believing that one has cancer, is loved by a famous person, or is being deceived by a spouse or lover. These patients do not have a thought disorder, and they are able to function socially.

Schizoaffective disorder. In schizoaffective disorder, symptoms of depression or mania coexist with those of schizophrenia. However, for the clinician to make the diagnosis, there must be a period during which the patient has only psychotic symptoms and no mood symptoms. Schizoaffective disorder has a better prognosis than schizophrenia but a poorer prognosis than mood disorders. Patients with schizophrenia may have mood symptoms, but generally the mood symptoms are of brief duration, are not prominent, and tend to occur only during the prodromal or residual phases.

■ EVALUATION

Consistent with the preceding discussion, the initial step in evaluating a patient who is exhibiting psychotic symptoms is to exclude an etiologic role for general medical conditions or substance use. This process assumes particular importance in patients with new-onset psychosis. A thorough clinical evaluation—including personal medical history, substance use history (including prescribed and over-the-counter medications), history of head trauma, family medical history, and medical review of systems—is mandatory. A systematic physical and neurological examination should be performed. During the mental status examination, impairments in orientation, fluctuations in awareness and consciousness, impaired recent memory, and the presence of nonauditory hallucinations point to a medical or substance-induced origin.

Routine laboratory tests may be helpful. These tests include a complete blood count, chemistry profile, thyroid function tests, urinalysis, urine drug screen, and venereal disease research laboratory (VDRL) testing. HIV testing may often be indicated. The choice of other tests should be guided by the patient's history and physical examination results; for example, computed tomography or magnetic resonance imaging scans of the head should be considered for patients who have a history of head trauma, for those who show neurological signs, or during the initial workup of patients with new-onset psychosis. If no medical or substance-use etiology is discovered and the psychotic symptoms persist, consultation with a psychiatrist may aid in the diagnostic process. A psychiatrist can confirm the absence of medical conditions or substances as etiologic factors and can evaluate patients for psychiatric conditions involving psychotic symptoms.

■ ROLE OF PRIMARY CARE PRACTITIONERS

Primary care practitioners may encounter patients who exhibit acute psychosis. Psychiatric consultation should be obtained to confirm the diagnosis; to evaluate the patient's potential for suicide, homicide, or violent behavior; to determine whether psychiatric hospitalization is indicated; and, if necessary, to assist with involuntary commitment (13). The psychiatrist can help develop a treatment plan and can aid in selecting a medication and dosage. Later, the psychiatrist can recommend specialized psychosocial treatments.

For the most part, patients will not present to outpatient clinics in a floridly psychotic manner. Instead, the primary care practitioner is likely to encounter patients who have chronic psychotic disorders, especially schizophrenia. In addition, families may bring in patients who have milder symptoms or who are in the earlier stages of psychotic decompensation. Patients who have chronic schizophrenia and related chronic psychotic disorders may receive most if not all of their care from primary care practitioners. As such, primary care practitioners are well positioned to provide a stable social contact for patients who often have few sustained interpersonal relationships and to offer supportive psychotherapy emphasizing adaptation to reality (13, 14).

Because primary care practitioners may get to know these patients over extended periods and become quite familiar with their baseline levels of symptoms and functioning, they will be able to detect when a relapse is imminent. Generally, patients will not volunteer that they are experiencing a recurrence of psychosis. The primary care practitioner must be vigilant and suspect incipient relapse when the patient's hygiene declines or his or her dress becomes slovenly, when the patient's thoughts become harder to follow or become more sparse, or when the patient fails to show up for an appointment. Patients should be questioned often about compliance with antipsychotic medication treatment regimens. Noncompliance is the most common cause of relapse and may relate to side effects, denial of illness, preference for psychosis over the rigors or boredom of reality, or other factors (14). Psychiatrists should be consulted to help manage a relapse or to discuss a change in medications.

Patients who have chronic psychotic conditions should have regularly scheduled appointments and screening examinations.

However, some patients are too impaired to keep appointments or to be compliant with medications and will come to the clinic only during emergencies (15). The primary care practitioner must recognize that patients who have chronic psychotic conditions may describe real physical complaints in a bizarre or idiosyncratic fashion (e.g., "snakes biting the inside of my stomach"). Thus genuine medical illness may be confused with delusional thinking (13).

The overall mortality rate for patients who have schizophrenia is approximately twice that for the general population. Most of this increased mortality is the result of deaths from respiratory and cardiovascular disorders. The contribution to this mortality rate of a sedentary lifestyle, heavy smoking, or obesity resulting from use of psychotropic drugs is not clear (16). Furthermore, approximately 10% of individuals with schizophrenia commit suicide (16).

Because patients may not be forthcoming, the primary care practitioner can ask indirect questions about symptoms. For instance, a chronically paranoid patient may be asked, "How are your neighbors? Are they still bothering you?" If patients ask whether the practitioner believes their delusions, an appropriate response would be "I'm not sure. I don't think I know enough about that [the delusional material] yet." The practitioner's manner should be friendly but not effusive. Beyond a handshake, the practitioner should not touch guarded patients except during physical examinations, and jokes should be avoided because patients may misinterpret them. Silences on the part of the patient should be accepted as part of the patient's relational style, although new silences in a previously garrulous individual may suggest a relapse (15).

■ GENERAL PRINCIPLES OF TREATMENT

Antipsychotic Drugs

Since the introduction of chlorpromazine (Thorazine) in the early 1950s, antipsychotic drugs have become the mainstay of treatment for a variety of psychotic conditions. Table 6–4 lists antipsychotic drugs available in the United States (17). The diphenylbutylpiperidine pimozide, approved for use in Tourette syndrome, is also a potent antipsychotic. The atypical antipsychotics are clozapine (Clozaril), risperidone (Risperdal), olanzapine (Zyprexa), and quetiapine (Seroquel). Treatment with these medications should be initiated only after consultation with a psychiatrist.

There are no well-established differences between specific antipsychotic drugs (with the exception of atypical agents). All traditional antipsychotics appear equally effective when administered in equipotent dosages. Haloperidol (Haldol) and fluphenazine (Prolixin), which are given in low milligram dosages, are considered high-potency antipsychotics. Conversely, chlorpromazine (Thorazine), thioridazine (Mellaril), and mesoridazine (Serentil), which are given in high milligram amounts, are considered low-potency antipsychotics. Low-potency agents have a reduced incidence of extrapyramidal side effects (EPS) but produce more sedation, orthostatic hypotension, and anticholinergic effects. High-potency antipsychotics are associated with less sedation, orthostatic hypotension, and anticholinergic effects, but they have a greater propensity to produce EPS. Drugs with intermediate potency—for example, loxapine (Loxitane), molindone (Moban), and perphenazine (Trilafon)—have a side-effect profile that lies between these two groups. Because equipotent doses of traditional antipsychotics are equally effective, the choice of medication is determined largely by the medication's side-effect profile. In general, treatment with high-potency antipsychotics is recommended. A primary care practitioner should try to master the use of one high-potency drug such as haloperidol and one low-potency drug such as thioridazine.

Treatment of Acute Psychosis

Acute psychosis may result from any of the psychiatric, medical, or substance-induced disorders discussed earlier in this chapter. Treatment should be managed by a psychiatrist. Most patients can be started on 2–5 mg of haloperidol orally or its equivalent two to

TABLE 6–4. **Antipsychotic drugs currently available in the United States**

Class and drug	Usual adult dosage (mg/day)	Sedative effect	Orthostatic hypotension	Anticholinergic effect	Incidence of extrapyramidal side effects
Phenothiazines					
Chlorpromazine	100–1,000	High	High	High	Low–moderate
Thioridazine	100–800	High	High	Very high	Low
Mesoridazine	50–400	High	High	High	Low
Perphenazine	8–64	Moderate	Moderate	Moderate	Moderate
Trifluoperazine	5–50	Low–moderate	Low	Low	High
Fluphenazine	2–30	Low	Low	Low	High
Thioxanthenes					
Thiothixene	5–50	Low–moderate	Low	Low	High
Chlorprothixene	100–600	High	High	High	Low–moderate
Butyrophenones					
Haloperidol	2–20	Low	Low	Low	High
Dibenzoxazepines					
Loxapine	20–200	Moderate	Moderate	Moderate	Moderate
Dihydroindolones					
Molindone	20–200	Moderate	Moderate	Moderate	Moderate

(continued)

TABLE 6–4. **Antipsychotic drugs currently available in the United States *(continued)***

Class and drug	Usual adult dosage (mg/day)	Sedative effect	Orthostatic hypotension	Anticholinergic effect	Incidence of extrapyramidal side effects
Diphenylbutylpiperidines					
Pimozide	2–10	Low	Low	Low	High
Dibenzodiazepines					
Clozapine	150–900	High	High	Very high	Very low
Benzisoxazoles					
Risperidone	2–10	Low	Moderate	Low	Low
Thienobenzopiazepines					
Olanzapine	5–20	Moderate	Low	Moderate	Very low–low
Dibenzothiazepines					
Quetiapine	250–500	Moderate	Moderate	Low	Very low–low
Long-acting injectables					
Fluphenazine decanoate	12.5–50 mg every 1–4 weeks				
Haloperidol decanoate	50–250 mg every 2–4 weeks				

three times per day. The uncontrollable patient may require more frequent dosing or the intramuscular route of administration early in treatment. Initially, divided doses reduce side effects and provide ongoing sedation. After about 1 week, the entire dosage may be given at bedtime. Continued agitation is best managed with the short-term use of adjunctive benzodiazepines. Anticholinergic medication (e.g., benztropine mesylate [Cogentin], 1–2 mg bid) should be initiated as prophylaxis against EPS in patients taking high-potency antipsychotic drugs or in those younger than 45 years. The dosage can be increased to an average oral target dosage of 10–20 mg haloperidol or its equivalent daily. No evidence indicates that higher dosages provide any advantage for the vast majority of patients; rather, higher dosages may lead to unnecessary side effects. A trial should last 4–6 weeks, because improvement with antipsychotics is a gradual process. In the elderly, lower dosages should be used with longer periods between dosage increases.

If the patient fails to respond, the initial drug should be replaced by a typical antipsychotic drug from a different class or an atypical antipsychotic other than clozapine. In view of its association with agranulocytosis, clozapine should probably be reserved for patients who have failed to respond to, or are intolerant of, typical antipsychotic drugs and other atypical agents. In addition, nonantipsychotic drugs have been used as augmenting agents in patients who respond poorly to antipsychotics. These alternative drugs include lithium, carbamazepine, propranolol, antidepressants, and benzodiazepines; these medications should also be used only after consultation with a psychiatrist.

Maintenance Antipsychotic Drug Treatment

The long-term use of antipsychotic drugs has been best studied in the treatment of schizophrenia. After a first episode of acute schizophrenia, antipsychotics should be continued for at least 1 year. After a second episode, they should be continued for at least 5 years. A history of relapse after an attempt at discontinuation of antipsychotics and the presence of continued symptoms are indications for maintenance treatment. Controlled clinical trials have demonstrated that more than 50% of schizophrenic patients not taking antipsychotic drugs relapse within 4–6 months, compared with 20% of patients who continue antipsychotic drug treatment (18). As with acute treatment, patients should receive the lowest antipsychotic dosage possible during maintenance, particularly in view of the risk of tardive dyskinesia (TD). Haloperidol and fluphenazine are available as long-acting decanoate esters for intramuscular injection. If the patient might be noncompliant, a depot preparation may be indicated. Average dosages are 12.5–50 mg fluphenazine decanoate every 1–4 weeks or 50–250 mg haloperidol decanoate every 2–4 weeks. Long-term antipsychotic drug treatment should be avoided in conditions other than schizophrenia.

■ SIDE EFFECTS OF ANTIPSYCHOTICS

Extrapyramidal Side Effects

Acute dystonic reactions are among the most dramatic and subjectively frightening side effects of antipsychotic drug therapy. They usually develop within hours or days of the start of treatment and are seen most commonly in young males. Acute dystonic reactions consist of muscle spasms typically involving the mouth, tongue, eyes, neck, and back. Fortunately, these symptoms are very responsive to intravenous or intramuscular treatment with anticholinergic agents such as benztropine mesylate 1–2 mg or diphenhydramine (Benadryl) 25–50 mg.

Akathisia involves an unpleasant sensation of motor restlessness felt most prominently in the legs and a corresponding difficulty sitting still. Patients may appear agitated and pace about the room. Akathisia typically occurs within the first 4 weeks of starting antipsychotic drug treatment and may develop after the first dose. It may be mistaken for anxiety or a worsening of psychosis and may be treated inappropriately with an increase in antipsychotic drug dosage. Anticholinergic agents appear relatively ineffective in relieving akathisia. Benzodiazepines may be helpful; however, the β-adrenergic blockers, particularly propranolol, appear to be the agents of choice.

Antipsychotic drug–induced Parkinsonism can have all the features of idiopathic Parkinson's disease, including bradykinesia, rigidity, and tremors. It has a gradual onset, typically developing over 2–4 weeks after the start of therapy, and is more common in the elderly. Treatment involves oral anticholinergic drugs or the dopamine agonist amantadine (Symmetrel).

Tardive Dyskinesia

TD is a persistent and potentially irreversible complication of treatment with antipsychotic drugs. This disorder rarely develops in patients who are exposed to antipsychotics for less than 3–6 months, although in the elderly it has been known to emerge after 1 month of treatment (11). TD is a syndrome of abnormal involuntary movements involving the musculature of the tongue, face, neck, trunk, or upper and lower extremities. Advancing age appears to be the most important risk factor for developing TD. Other risk factors may include female gender, diabetes, high antipsychotic drug dosage, long duration of exposure, history of acute EPS, and a diagnosis of mood disorder. The typical antipsychotics appear to cause TD with equal frequency. Clozapine, however, seems to have little or no risk of causing this disorder. It is not yet clear to what extent the newer atypical agents also have a decreased association with TD. For most patients, TD is not progressive and tends to stabilize or improve despite continued treatment. Furthermore, most cases of TD are mild, although some patients develop a severe and disabling form of the disorder.

Patients should be evaluated for abnormal movements at the start of treatment and on a regular basis thereafter. If a patient develops TD, he or she should be referred to a psychiatrist to determine whether the antipsychotic dosage can be decreased. A psychiatrist may also decide, at that point, to use one of the newer agents. If treatment with antipsychotics can be stopped, TD remits in 5%–40% of all cases and in 50%–90% of mild cases (11). In view of the likelihood of relapse, however, most patients with chronic schizophrenia should continue taking antipsychotic drugs. When continued treatment is elected, an attempt should be made to reduce the dosage. If TD is severe, a switch to clozapine or possibly a newer atypical agent should be considered.

Neuroleptic Malignant Syndrome

Neuroleptic malignant syndrome (NMS) is a rare but potentially fatal syndrome that occurs in patients who are taking neuroleptics. Core features include hyperthermia, muscle rigidity, mental status changes, and autonomic dysfunction. NMS usually occurs within 4 weeks after the start of treatment. Hyperthermia usually develops concomitantly with or shortly after rigidity. Impairment of mental status may result in confusion, stupor, coma, and catatonia. Autonomic dysfunction may be manifested by labile or elevated blood pressure, pallor, diaphoresis, incontinence, tachycardia, and tachypnea. Patients with NMS are very ill and require hospitalization.

Common laboratory abnormalities in NMS include elevated levels of serum creatine phosphokinase and other muscle enzymes and leukocytosis. Myonecrosis may lead to myoglobinuria and renal failure. Treatment should include a psychiatric consultation consisting primarily of early recognition, discontinuation of antipsychotics, and institution of meticulous supportive care. Use of dopamine agonists such as bromocriptine (Parlodel) or the direct-acting muscle relaxant dantrolene (Dantrium) should be considered in more severe or prolonged cases.

Other Side Effects

All antipsychotics can cause seizures, particularly at higher dosages. Low-potency agents carry the greatest risk. Molindone may have an especially infrequent association with seizures. Anticholinergic effects such as dry mouth, blurred vision, decreased sweating, urinary hesitancy, and constipation are also more common with low-potency antipsychotics. Anticholinergic drugs used to treat EPS exert additive effects. Untreated narrow-angle glaucoma is an absolute contraindication to anticholinergic drug use, and prostatic hypertrophy is a relative contraindication. More severe peripheral anticholinergic effects include urinary retention and ileus. Central nervous system effects include impairment in memory and concentration, which may progress to agitation and delirium, especially in the elderly.

The most frequent cardiovascular complication of antipsychotics is orthostatic hypotension, which relates to α-adrenergic blockade and is most common with low-potency drugs. Thioridazine, mesoridazine, and pimozide may slow cardiac conduction, prolonging the corrected QT interval. Ventricular tachycardia may occur during overdosages and possibly at therapeutic dosages (19). High-potency agents such as haloperidol are preferred in patients with known heart disease.

Hyperprolactinemia occurs with typical antipsychotics and potentially results in amenorrhea in women and gynecomastia and galactorrhea in both genders. In addition, all antipsychotics cause weight gain, with the probable exception of molindone. Antipsychotics predispose patients to heat stroke by blocking hypothalamic thermoregulatory mechanisms. Sexual effects may include decreased libido, change in the quality of orgasm, and anorgasmia in both genders, and delayed ejaculation and priapism in men. Thioridazine may cause painful retrograde ejaculation.

Eye effects include granular deposits in the lens and cornea during long-term chlorpromazine treatment, although these deposits rarely impair vision, and retinitis pigmentosa during thioridazine treatment at dosages above 800 mg/day, which can lead to visual impairment or blindness. Skin effects may include allergic rashes resolving with drug discontinuation. In addition, all antipsychotics, particularly low-potency agents, may be associated with photosensitivity resulting in severe sunburn. Furthermore, long-term treatment with low-potency agents can cause a blue-gray discoloration of the skin.

Hepatic effects center around cholestatic jaundice, which may develop as a hypersensitivity reaction during the first 2 months of treatment. It is associated primarily with chlorpromazine, although it has been observed occasionally with several other phenothiazines. The most important hematologic effect is agranulocytosis, a life-threatening complication that develops in only 1–5 in 10,000 patients taking antipsychotic drugs other than clozapine. It is seen primarily during the first 2 months of treatment and is associated with low-potency agents. Patients should be advised to report signs of infection such as sore throat or fever. As a general rule, antipsychotic drugs should be used only if absolutely necessary during pregnancy; however, no clear association exists between congenital malformations and antipsychotic drug treatment (19). Because antipsychotics are secreted in milk, mothers taking antipsychotics should not breast-feed.

■ ATYPICAL AGENTS

Clozapine is the prototype of a new group of atypical antipsychotics, distinguished from traditional drugs by their minimal production of EPS and their enhanced efficacy. Clozapine causes little or no TD (20) and is also effective in treating negative symptoms. Candidates for clozapine use include patients with psychosis that is refractory to treatment with traditional drugs, patients intolerant of EPS, and patients with severe TD.

A major drawback of clozapine therapy is agranulocytosis, which occurs in roughly 1% of patients taking the medication. Therefore, patients must have weekly white blood cell monitoring. More than 95% of cases of agranulocytosis occur within the first 6 months of treatment, and women may be at higher risk (19). Stopping treatment with clozapine leads to recovery in most cases (21). Seizures are common when dosages higher than 600 mg/day are used. Other side effects include hypersalivation, sedation, tachycardia, orthostatic hypotension, weight gain, and anticholinergic effects.

Risperidone was the second atypical agent introduced. It is at least as potent and antipsychotic as haloperidol (22). It, too, is less likely to cause EPS than traditional agents and appears to be effective in controlling negative symptoms. The most effective dosage is 2–6 mg/day. However, if the dosage is increased beyond 6 mg/day, the risk of developing EPS increases. It is not known whether risperidone will be effective in patients with psychosis that is refractory to treatment with traditional antipsychotics or whether it will have a reduced association with TD. Risperidone has been used with some success in the elderly. Its side effects include orthostatic hypotension (particularly at the start of treatment), nausea, weight gain, headache, and ejaculatory disturbances.

Olanzapine was the third atypical agent introduced. Like risperidone, it is at least as effective as haloperidol in treating positive symptoms and is more effective in treating negative symptoms (23). Olanzapine has a low risk of causing EPS. Furthermore, it appears to have a reduced association with TD compared with traditional drugs. The usual effective dosage is 10–20 mg/day. It is not known how effective olanzapine will be for patients with treatment-refractory psychosis. Side effects include orthostatic hypotension, weight gain, drowsiness, constipation, and dry mouth.

The most recent atypical antipsychotic to be introduced is quetiapine. This agent is at least as effective as haloperidol for positive symptoms and appears to have superior efficacy for negative symptoms (24). Quetiapine therapy is generally initiated at 75 mg/day in divided doses and may be titrated up to 750 mg/day. The optimal dosage appears to be 250–500 mg/day. Quetiapine has a very low tendency to cause EPS across its dosage range. One potential disadvantage of the current preparation of quetiapine is its rather short half-life, suggesting that twice-daily dosing is necessary. Side effects include drowsiness, orthostatic hypotension, weight gain, and headache. Quetiapine does not appear to have significant anticholinergic effects. As with risperidone and olanzapine, it is unknown whether quetiapine is as useful as clozapine in patients with psychosis that is refractory to treatment with traditional antipsychotic medications.

CONCLUSION

Psychosis can occur in a variety of disorders. The initial evaluation should include screening for medical conditions or substances as etiologic agents. If none are identified, then schizophrenia and the other psychotic disorders should be considered in the differential diagnosis. Consultation with a psychiatrist can help in clarifying the diagnosis and establishing a treatment plan. A variety of antipsychotic agents are available, including four atypical agents introduced in the 1990s. Most psychotic disorders are chronic and will require continuous and thorough follow-up.

REFERENCES

1. Caine ED, Grossman H, Lyness JM: Delirium, dementia, and amnestic and other cognitive disorders and mental disorders due to a general medical condition, in Comprehensive Textbook of Psychiatry, 6th Edition. Edited by Kaplan HI, Sadock BJ. Baltimore, MD, Williams & Wilkins, 1995, pp 705–754
2. Slater E, Beard AW: The schizophrenia-like psychoses of epilepsy: psychiatric aspects. Br J Psychiatry 109:95–150, 1963
3. Cummings JL: Organic psychoses: delusional disorder and secondary mania. Psychiatr Clin North Am 9:293–312, 1986
4. Thomas CS, Szabadi E: Paranoid psychosis as the first presentation of a fulminating lethal case of AIDS. Br J Psychiatry 151:693–695, 1987
5. Wilson WH, Jefferson JW: Thyroid disease, behavior, and psychopharmacology. Psychosomatics 26:481–492, 1985
6. Estroff TW, Gold MS: Medication-induced and toxin-induced psychiatric disorders, in Medical Mimics of Psychiatric Disorders. Edited by Estroff I, Gold MS. Washington, DC, American Psychiatric Press, 1986, pp 163–198
7. Drugs that cause psychiatric symptoms. Med Lett Drugs Ther 35:65–70, 1993
8. Hurlbut KM: Drug-induced psychoses. Emerg Med Clin North Am 9:31–52, 1991
9. Beeder AB, Millman RB: Patients with psychopathology, in Substance Abuse: a Comprehensive Textbook, 3rd Edition. Edited by Lowison JH, Ruiz P, Millman RB, et al. Baltimore, MD, Williams & Wilkins, 1997, pp 551–563

10. Gunderson JG, Phillips KA: Personality disorders, in Comprehensive Textbook of Psychiatry, 6th Edition. Edited by Kaplan HI, Sadock BJ. Baltimore, MD, Williams & Wilkins, 1995, pp 1425–1461
11. American Psychiatric Association: Diagnostic and Statistical Manual of Mental Disorders, 4th Edition. Washington, DC, American Psychiatric Association, 1994
12. Karno M, Norquist GS: Schizophrenia: epidemiology, in Comprehensive Textbook of Psychiatry, 6th Edition. Edited by Kaplan HI, Sadock BJ. Baltimore, MD, Williams & Wilkins, 1995, pp 902–910
13. Dubovsky SL, Weissberg MP: Clinical Psychiatry in Primary Care. Baltimore, MD, Williams & Wilkins, 1986
14. Dubovsky SL: Concise Guide to Clinical Psychiatry. Washington, DC, American Psychiatric Press, 1988
15. Burns T, Kendrick T: Schizophrenia, in Psychiatry and General Practice Today. Edited by Pullen I, Wilkinson G, Wright A, et al. Glasgow, Scotland, Bell & Bain, 1994, pp 194–208
16. Allbeck P: Schizophrenia: a life-shortening disease. Psychopharmacol Bull 15:81–89, 1989
17. Van Kammen DP, Marder SR: Dopamine receptor antagonists, in Comprehensive Textbook of Psychiatry, 6th Edition. Edited by Kaplan HI, Sadock BJ. Baltimore, MD, Williams & Wilkins, 1995, pp 1987–2022
18. Davis JM: Overview: maintenance therapy in psychiatry, I: schizophrenia. Am J Psychiatry 132:1237–1245, 1975
19. Hyman SE, Arana GW, Rosenbaum JF: Handbook of Psychiatric Drug Therapy, 3rd Edition. Boston, MA, Little, Brown, 1995
20. Lieberman JA: Pharmacotherapy for patients with first-episode, acute, and refractory schizophrenia. Psychiatric Annals 26:515–518, 1996
21. Meltzer HY: Predictors of response to clozapine. Psychiatric Annals 26:385–389, 1996
22. Marder S, Meiback RC: Risperidone in the treatment of schizophrenia. Am J Psychiatry 151:825–835, 1994
23. Beasley CM Jr, Tollefson G, Tran P, et al: Olanzapine versus placebo and haloperidol: acute phase results of the North American double-blind olanzapine trial. Neuropsychopharmacology 14:111–123, 1996
24. Arvanitis LA, Miller BG: Multiple fixed doses of "Seroquel" (quetiapine) in patients with acute exacerbation of schizophrenia: a comparison with haloperidol and placebo. The Seroquel Trial 13 Study Group. Biol Psychiatry 42:233–246, 1997

7

DIFFICULT DOCTOR-PATIENT RELATIONSHIPS

Michael F. Gliatto, M.D.

For the most part, physicians and patients in primary care practice form a relationship they expect to be enduring and satisfying. In this chapter, I address relationships in which a sense of mutual satisfaction does not occur. The emphasis is on the physician's perspective, and some basic suggestions are given for working with all patients. Although physicians are mentioned exclusively, this chapter applies to all practitioners in a primary care setting.

Physicians find 10% of relationships with patients to be frustrating (1). Similarly, in a study of patients who frequently use ambulatory services, physicians labeled 37% of the patients as frustrating (2). Three key variables, either alone or in combination, appear to cause physicians to think of patients as problematic (3, 4):

1. The patient is seen as having a *difficult style.*
2. There is *no certain diagnosis.*
3. The patient's problems are thought to be *psychosocial.*

■ PATIENT VARIABLES

Styles

For the purposes of this chapter, I define *style* as a set of behaviors or traits that affect the doctor-patient relationship and, hence, the treatment. Style is not synonymous with character, personality, or personality disorder. Styles have been typified by various writers as dependent, angry or demanding, suffering, self-destructive, and somatizing (1, 5–7). These styles are more akin to stereotypes, and no one can be reduced to the adjectives *dependent* or *angry*. Likewise, an abrasive style does not imply that the patient does not have structural or physiological abnormalities. Rather, the concept of styles is used to facilitate understanding of how patients react to illnesses, and that understanding is used in designing individual treatment plans.

Dependent. Patients with a dependent style are overtly needy. Physicians like to help them initially but then tire of them (5).

Demanding. Patients with a demanding style are covertly needy. Rather than state their needs, they demand, argue, and try to dictate treatment. Physicians, in turn, feel anxious, belittled, and angry (6).

Suffering. Patients with a suffering style unconsciously want to feel anguished and do not expect relief from their symptoms. Pain and suffering are ways to cement the relationship with the physician (6).

Self-destructive. Patients with a self-destructive style are noncompliant and often abuse substances. They may see a physician when they feel acutely ill and may stay in treatment briefly but then do not follow up. Physicians feel hopeless and frustrated when working with these patients.

Somatizing. Somatizing is not the same as somatization disorder. Patients who use a somatizing style express psychological phenomena in bodily terms. For example, instead of feeling angry or sad, a patient may complain of a headache. This use of physical symptoms is unconscious and is not for gain—for example, to get out of work (8).

These styles can be demonstrated in the following cases:

> Mrs. A. is a 48-year-old divorced woman who works as a secretary at the local high school. She has had complaints of abdominal bloating, constipation, and pain for the past 6 months.
>
> Mrs. A. always comes in early for her appointments, takes her medications, and frequently asks her doctor for advice about what to eat. After her mother, with whom she lives, has a stroke and is left bedridden, Mrs. A. complains of increasing abdominal pain. Her physical examination is unrevealing, but the pain persists. She becomes annoyed when her doctor tells her the pain is "in your head."

> Mr. B. is a 75-year-old retired businessman who, since having a heart attack 2 years earlier, is preoccupied with measuring his salt and fluid intake. When he begins to experience dyspnea when climbing stairs, he demands that his generalist refer him to a cardiologist. The generalist recommends increasing the dosage of Mr. B.'s diuretic. Mr. B. sighs with annoyance and leaves.
>
> Mr. B. begins to call the generalist's office daily, saying that his weight is increasing and that his shoes no longer fit. Exasperated, the generalist refers him to a local cardiologist. Mr. B. asks the cardiologist, "Don't you think I need a catheterization?" The cardiologist also recommends the use of diuretics.
>
> Mr. B. decides to see another generalist in town. He tells the new doctor that his previous doctor was inept and complains that the cardiologist did not do a thorough exam.

It could be said that Mrs. A. is an example of the somatizing patient and Mr. B. is a example of the angry, demanding patient. However, Mrs. A. may also demonstrate elements of the suffering style. Likewise, Mr. B. somatizes. These styles were not evident at the onset of their illnesses but became manifest only after the symptoms became more severe; in some patients, the style is apparent at the first office visit.

These cases also describe behaviors that physicians attribute to so-called difficult patients. These behaviors include the following (8):

- Missing appointments
- Calling the office frequently
- Visiting after hours or in emergency rooms
- Failing to respond to conservative measures and reassurance
- Denying the presence of psychosocial problems

Difficult patients are more likely to be widowed, divorced, or unemployed than are nondifficult patients, and they tend to be older and less educated than the latter group (2, 9).

Table 7–1 offers treatment guidelines for the five styles discussed in this chapter. Additional recommendations, including those pertaining to the cases provided in this section, are given later in the chapter in the Suggestions for Treatment section.

Uncertain Diagnoses and Psychosocial Problems

Physicians are annoyed by patients who have disorders for which the diagnosis is uncertain or by those who exhibit psychosocial problems. In 25%–50% of visits to primary care clinics, no serious cause is found to account for the patients' symptoms, but rather the visits are precipitated by psychosocial reasons (8).

According to Barsky (10), there are four psychosocial reasons that patients see doctors:

1. *Life stressors.* Divorce, death or illness of family members, unemployment, and a host of other stressors lead people to identify themselves as patients and to seek medical attention. Patients find that seeing a physician on a regular basis alleviates the stress to some extent.
2. *Treatment of psychiatric disorders.* Patients with psychiatric disorders are more apt to see a generalist than a psychiatrist, as will be discussed below.
3. *Loneliness.* Appointments with doctors are a form of social contact.
4. *Education.* Patients want to learn about symptoms, illnesses, and treatment.

TABLE 7–1. **Treatment recommendations for different patient styles**

Style	Treatment recommendations
Dependent	Schedule frequent appointments
	Set appropriate limits concerning use of emergency rooms or calling between appointments
	Try to maintain an optimal level of functioning in the patient
Demanding	Schedule frequent appointments
	Do not question the patient's sense of entitlement
	Do not try to "win" discussions with the patient (i.e., do not try to show the patient that he or she is misguided or incorrect, unless treatment is threatened)
	Set appropriate limits concerning scheduling appointments or use of diagnostic testing (i.e., the patient cannot expect an immediate appointment nor can he or she demand inappropriate tests)
	Inform the patient of all treatment decisions, side effects of medications, prognostications, and so on; supply literature
Suffering	Do not expect a cure
	Schedule frequent appointments
	Focus on one symptom complex at a time
Self-destructive	Address the most acute problem at the time of presentation (e.g., tracheobronchitis in an emphysematous patient who smokes, endocarditis in a patient who abuses heroin, acidosis in a noncompliant diabetic patient)
	Do not issue ultimatums
	Do not expect that you will change the patient; expect a series of sudden appearances and disappearances
Somatizing	Schedule frequent appointments
	Limit diagnostic tests
	Maintain an optimal level of functioning in the patient

As with the concept of styles, more than one reason may be involved in any particular doctor visit. Regarding the cases provided earlier, one can surmise that Mrs. A. and Mr. B. had expectations that their contact with their physicians would alleviate the stress in their lives, that they could discuss ideas with their physicians, and that they would learn something about their symptoms. They also may have had psychiatric disorders.

Sixty percent of patients with psychiatric disorders receive psychiatric care from generalists (10). This high percentage may have several explanations, including lack of access to a psychiatrist, feelings of shame associated with seeing a psychiatrist, and the obfuscation of psychiatric symptoms by somatic complaints or chronic medical illnesses (11). It follows then that some so-called difficult patients will have an underlying psychiatric disorder (1, 7). Unfortunately, such patients often resist psychiatric referral. Another aggravating factor is that patients seen in primary care clinics often do not meet the criteria for disorders as delineated in DSM-IV (12). Instead, patients have a mixture of symptoms that are part of the affective, anxiety, somatoform, and substance abuse disorders (11, 13, 14). Mrs. A. and Mr. B. may have had some symptoms consistent with a major depressive disorder, a somatoform pain disorder, or an anxiety disorder.

■ EFFECT OF THESE VARIABLES ON THE DOCTOR-PATIENT RELATIONSHIP

What seems to distress physicians about difficult styles, uncertain diagnoses, and psychosocial problems is that these factors disturb physicians' sense that they are using their skills effectively to help people. The expectation that a process will occur, beginning with the interview, leading to a diagnosis and treatment plan, and ending with a mutual sense of accomplishment between patient and physician, is not realized (4). Instead, physicians become frustrated because they feel they have neither the time nor the expertise to handle psychosocial problems, they question their competence or the patient's reliability if a diagnosis is not found, or they develop an active dislike of the patient.

Thus far, the focus has been on the physician's perspective. However, to view all problems as the patient's doing is perilous, and it probably makes more sense to consider difficult doctor-patient relationships rather than difficult patients (4). What does the physician contribute to the difficulties in the relationship? Extensive literature does not exist on physician styles, but one could posit that physicians who are uncomfortable with ambiguities, chronicity, or the complexity of patients' personalities may be unhappy in primary care medical practice.

Physicians must try to improve relationships with patients once difficulties arise because patient anger is as strong a motivating force as physician negligence in initiating a malpractice suit (1). Maintenance of a sound doctor-patient relationship has economic benefits in that fewer unnecessary laboratory tests or procedures may be ordered. Also, by virtue of the physician's professionalism, it is the physician's responsibility, not the patient's, to attempt to correct whatever has gone awry in the doctor-patient relationship (4).

■ SUGGESTIONS FOR TREATMENT

This section contains suggestions for maintaining the doctor-patient relationship (see Table 7–2 for a summary). They are by no means exhaustive. Most of them apply to initial visits and some can be considered preventive in that they screen for future problems. It takes 5–10 minutes to ask these questions, but doing so can save hours later on.

Initial Visit(s)

1. Give the patient time to answer the question "How can I help you?" Two minutes is sufficient; after that, you can be more directive, but you should use a mixture of open- and close-ended questions. While the patient speaks, do a mental status exami-

TABLE 7–2. **Suggestions for working with patients**
Expect a long-term relationship
Give the patient time to explain symptoms
Concentrate on the patient's most troublesome complaint
Do not separate the physical from the psychosocial
Ask about previous treatments and about relationships with other doctors
Screen for psychiatric disorders
Conduct a physical examination
Ascertain treatment goals
Do not commit yourself to a diagnosis prematurely
Schedule frequent appointments
Educate the patient
Set appropriate limits
Know your own limitations

nation, particularly taking notice of the patient's appearance, mood, affect, behavior, and thought process.

2. If the patient has multiple complaints, ask him or her which one is most bothersome and focus on that one. Tell the patient that you will ask about other complaints on a subsequent visit. By doing so, you are letting the patient know that you are expecting a relationship to develop beginning with the first visit.
3. Do not separate the physical from the psychosocial. After the patient describes the symptom, ask, "How does the symptom get in the way of your daily life? How is your family getting along now that you have this symptom?" Had Mrs. A. been asked this question, the physician could have learned more about the possible connection between her stomach pain and her caring for her mother. Bringing up psychosocial issues after diagnostic testing has been completed may make the patient think that you do not believe that the symptoms are real; the patient then may become angry (15).
4. Listen to how the patient describes symptoms. Vague or personalized descriptions or those involving multiple organ systems suggest the somatization style (16).

5. Ask the patient about previous treatments and what worked or did not work. Asking about relationships with previous physicians can be awkward. However, you can ask, "What other physicians have you seen? How was Dr. X. helpful?" Knowing about other doctors will give you some idea of what to expect in the future. For example, a patient who had trouble with Dr. X. may also have trouble with you. Mr. B. had problems with two of the doctors mentioned; one can assume that he may also become disillusioned with the third.
6. Conduct a physical examination even if you doubt that it will be enlightening. The performance of the examination has its own reassuring qualities (17).
7. Ask the patient about his or her expectations and goals. This issue is somewhat complicated and may have to be clarified over a series of visits. Several questions can be used to elicit this information, including "What worries you most about this symptom?" "Was there something that I forgot to ask you about or something else you would like me to know?" and "What sorts of things were you hoping would be accomplished today?" If a patient is worried that his or her pain is from an underlying malignancy, and nothing in the workup suggests it, you can reassure the patient accordingly. If a patient is expecting a cure for rheumatoid arthritis or another chronic disease, you can help the patient set more realistic goals. The answers to these questions can also indicate any psychosocial reasons involved in the visit.

In terms of the cases provided earlier, what Mr. B. hoped to accomplish apparently was to obtain a catheterization; he may have also hoped unrealistically that his symptoms would disappear as quickly as possible. In terms of setting goals, the generalist could have defined a specific period for increasing the diuretic dosage, such as 2 weeks, before consulting the cardiologist. With Mrs. A., the pain likely may persist despite conservative measures. Rather than dismiss the pain as psychosomatic, however, it would be best for the physician to reassure her that nothing alarming was found on the examination and that the physician will see her frequently to monitor her progress and to maximize her daily functioning.

8. Ask screening questions for psychiatric disorders, particularly substance abuse disorders, major depressive disorder, generalized anxiety disorder, and somatization disorder. These questions need to be asked early in the course of working with a patient. If they are asked later, the patient may find them offensive, which will make a psychiatric referral that much harder.
9. If you are unsure of the diagnosis, do not commit yourself to any one diagnosis (7, 16). You can tell a patient what the diagnosis is not, especially if he or she has unrealistic worries about a particular diagnosis (17). You may say, "I don't know what this symptom is part of yet, but I will see you again and it may take several visits before the diagnosis is clear. I can tell you now, based on what you told me and what I've noticed on the physical exam, that this weakness in your arm is not from another stroke." If the doctor-patient relationship is well established, unexplained symptoms may resolve with time and no specific treatment other than watchful waiting.

Later Visits

1. Depending on what the patient's insurance policy allows, schedule regular appointments, even if no procedures or tests are planned. The relationship with the patient is as much a part of the treatment as are diagnostic studies (16).
2. Appropriate limits need to be set when various behaviors appear. If a patient asks to be seen more frequently than you deem necessary, remind the patient that you will see him or her as regularly as you can and for specific time periods (e.g., 15 minutes) but that the demands of your practice prevent you from scheduling more frequent appointments. If the patient comes between appointments, for example, if the managed care plan has a minimal or no copayment, remind the patient of

your agreement regarding regular visits and see him or her for several minutes only. What is not taken care of at that point can be addressed at the next scheduled appointment.

If a patient calls you frequently, tell the patient that because you are very busy with other patients, you cannot always return calls promptly. Office personnel can remind the patient that nonemergency calls are returned at specific times—for example, from 12:00 P.M. to 1:00 P.M. or after 5:00 P.M. It is a mistake to ignore the patient's calls altogether. An alternative is to suggest that the patient keep a diary of his or her symptoms or concerns and that the diary entries be discussed briefly at each visit.

If a patient sees other physicians without your knowledge or visits emergency rooms unnecessarily, inform the patient of your referral policy and tell him or her that seeing multiple physicians makes treatment confusing and can actually be harmful if the care is not coordinated by one physician. This issue should become less of a problem as managed care creates more integrated systems (8).

Similarly, limits should be placed on threatening or seductive behavior, noncompliance with medications, missed appointments, requests for controlled medications, or use of substances.

3. Coordination of care between psychiatrists and generalists reduces health care costs and increases patient satisfaction (18). A referral to a psychiatrist should be made only after the referral is discussed thoroughly with the patient. The patient may, of course, refuse. If the situation is not urgent, then you should wait and try again later. If the psychiatric consultation takes place, schedule a visit with the patient soon thereafter to learn what the patient thought about the consultation; this will reassure him or her that you will continue as the primary doctor and that care is not to be transferred entirely to the psychiatrist.

4. Educate the patient about the connection between stress and the onset or aggravation of symptoms. The patient should also be taught how to evaluate multiple symptoms and how to determine which need attention and which can wait until the next scheduled appointment (8). Nursing staff can help with this education and also with answering questions over the telephone. Such instruction would have been helpful to Mrs. A.
5. Know your own limits. If you find a patient particularly irksome, discuss the situation with a colleague who may be able to help you change or control your feelings toward the patient. You may also find patients whom you dislike no matter what you do and that your feelings interfere with your ability to be objective and to help these patients. It is best to recognize this situation and refer such patients to a colleague (7).

■ CONCLUSION

The suggestions provided in this chapter are meant to be guidelines only. Because of human individuality, problems that develop between doctors and patients can be corrected in multiple ways. The point to remember is that the doctor-patient relationship is an intrinsic part of the treatment, that it begins with the initial visit, and that it requires continuous scrutiny on the physician's part in order for it to be effective for both parties. Despite what happens between doctors and patients as they work together, it remains true, as Tolstoy said, that patients feel a "moral need" for doctors and that doctors "satisf[y] the eternal human need for hope of relief, for sympathetic action, which is felt in the presence of suffering" (19).

■ REFERENCES

1. Schwenk TL, Romano SE: Managing the difficult physician-patient relationship. Am Fam Physician 46:1503–1509, 1992
2. Lin EHB, Katon W, Von Korff M, et al: Frustrating patients: physician and patient perspectives among distressed high users of medical services. J Gen Intern Med 6:241–246, 1991

3. Crutcher JE, Bass MJ: The difficult patient and the troubled physician. J Fam Pract 11:933–938, 1980
4. Schwenk TL, Marquez JT, Lefever RD, et al: Physician and patient determinants in difficult physician-patient relationships. J Fam Pract 28:59–63, 1989
5. Groves JE: Taking care of the hateful patient. N Engl J Med 298:883–887, 1978
6. Kahana RJ, Bibring GL: Personality types in medical management, in Psychiatry and Medical Practice in a General Hospital. Edited by Zinberg NE. New York, International Universities Press, 1964, pp 108–123
7. Nesheim R: Caring for patients who are not easy to like. Postgrad Med 72:255–266, 1982
8. Barsky AJ, Borus JF: Somatization and medicalization in the era of managed care. JAMA 274:1931–1934, 1995
9. John C, Schwenk TL, Roi LD, et al: Medical care and demographic characteristics of 'difficult' patients. J Fam Pract 24:607–610, 1987
10. Barksy AJ: Hidden reasons some patients visit doctors. Ann Intern Med 94:492–498, 1981
11. Katon W, Von Korff M, Lin E, et al: Distressed high utilizers of medical care: DSM-III-R diagnoses and treatment needs. Gen Hosp Psychiatry 12:355–362, 1990
12. American Psychiatric Association: Diagnostic and Statistical Manual of Mental Disorders, 4th Edition. Washington, DC, American Psychiatric Association, 1994
13. Barrett JE, Barrett JA, Oxman TE, et al: The prevalence of psychiatric disorders in a primary care practice. Arch Gen Psychiatry 45:1100–1106, 1998
14. Schurman RA, Kramer PD, Mitchell JB: The hidden mental network: treatment of mental illness by nonpsychiatrist physicians. Arch Gen Psychiatry 42:89–94, 1985
15. Lennard-Jones JE: Functional gastrointestinal disorders. N Engl J Med 308:431–435, 1983
16. Drossman DA: The problem patient: evaluation and care of medical patients with psychosocial disturbances. Ann Intern Med 88:366–372, 1978
17. Sapira J: Reassurance therapy: what to say to symptomatic patients with benign diseases. Ann Intern Med 77:603–604, 1972

18. Smith GR, Monson RA, Ray DC: Psychiatric consultation in somatization disorder: a randomized controlled study. N Engl J Med 314: 1407–1413, 1986
19. Tolstoy L: War and Peace (1869). Translated by Edmunds R. Middlesex, England, Penguin, 1978, p 777

8

SEXUAL DISORDERS

Mary F. Morrison, M.D.
Antonio Fernando, M.D.
Monica Bishop, B.A.

Sexual function is influenced strongly by one's gender identity, self-esteem, and personal relationships and by the moral values of one's culture. Sexual problems are common; however, few patients will seek care primarily for a sexual complaint, and such complaints are recorded infrequently in the problem lists on patients' charts. In this chapter, we define healthy sexual function and summarize the nosology and epidemiology of sexual disorders. We also address clinical issues such as the taking of a sexual history, important aspects of the physical examination in diagnosing sexual dysfunction, and medications that impair sexual function. Finally, we describe current knowledge of specific sexual disorders, including their etiology and treatment.

■ HEALTHY SEXUAL FUNCTION

Healthy sexual activity and functioning may involve fantasies; masturbation; and interactions with a significant other, such as hugging, cuddling, fondling, oral and manual stimulation, intercourse, and other sexual behaviors. The complete sexual response cycle consists of four phases: appetitive, excitement, orgasmic, and resolution (1). The appetitive phase involves sexual fantasies and a desire for sexual activity. During the excitement phase, physiological changes occur. Women experience pelvic vasocongestion, swelling of the external genitalia, and vaginal lubrication. Men experience penile tumescence and erection. Orgasm is the peak of sexual pleasure with release of sexual tension and rhythmic contraction of the pelvic organs. Men have contractions in the prostate, seminal vesicles, and urethra that result in the emission of semen (1). In women, contractions occur in the vaginal wall and uterus. Men are temporarily refractory to further erection and orgasm, but women can respond almost immediately and can have multiple orgasms.

Sexual function involves the brain, the spinal cord, the pelvic nerves, and the integrity of the end organs: the penis in men and the clitoris and the vaginal area in women. Normal sexual functioning from arousal to resolution is a complex process requiring the interplay of the vascular and endocrine systems, in addition to the central and peripheral nervous systems. Lubrication is thought to be controlled parasympathetically, whereas vaginal blood flow and ejaculation are mediated sympathetically (2). The neurotransmitters dopamine and serotonin are involved in sexual functioning; the former is excitatory and the latter inhibitory. The hormone testosterone is important for libido in both men and women.

■ EVALUATION

Sexual dysfunction is a common problem in the general population. Examination of 23 studies of community samples showed a current prevalence of 5%–10% for inhibited female orgasm, 4%–9% for male erectile disorder, 4%–10% for inhibited male orgasm, and 36%–38% for premature ejaculation (3).

Patients with a variety of illnesses commonly seen in the primary care setting complain of sexual dysfunction. These illnesses include hypertension, peripheral vascular disease, diabetes, stroke, myocardial infarction, seizure disorder, end-stage renal disease, and multiple sclerosis (4–7).

Patient History

The primary care practitioner plays a vital role in the diagnosis and treatment of sexual dysfunctions. In some cases, the practitioner is familiar with both sexual partners. The practitioner is also generally the only trusted medical consultant of many patients. Practitioners who routinely take a sexual history reported that 33.3% of their patients had some type of sexual concern, whereas those who do not include such a history reported that only 9.5% had a sexual concern (8). Clearly, patients are reluctant to volunteer concerns about sexual dysfunction, and direct inquiry by the physician is important in ascertaining whether a problem exists. The practitioner's attitude toward sexuality as a component of overall health is key to the proper screening and management of sexual dysfunction. The practitioner should obtain the sexual inventory in a way that is accepting and supportive of the patient's complaints, difficulties, habits, and practices.

When is the appropriate time for the physician to ask a patient about sexual function? A good practice is to incorporate the questions into the review of reproductive and urological systems. Patients are likely to feel more comfortable speaking about sexual problems when they are fully clothed in a consultation room than when they are wearing a hospital gown on the examining table. Vocabulary used should be based on cultural, ethnic, and educational considerations, and offensive language should not be used. Some patients may not be informed about sexual function or their own anatomy. The practitioner should assess the patient's level of knowledge and not assume understanding. The practitioner can assess for the presence of a sexual dysfunction by asking the six questions listed in Table 8–1 (9).

A positive response to one of the questions in Table 8–1 necessitates further inquiry. The following four questions should then be asked (9):

1. When did the symptoms begin?
2. Are they associated with any illness, surgery, physical deformity, or medication use?
3. Is the complaint or dysfunction intermittent or continuous?
4. Have you undergone any previous evaluations or treatments?

TABLE 8–1. **Screening tool for sexual dysfunction**

1. Have you noticed an increase or decrease in sexual desire and enjoyment?
2. Are you able to achieve and maintain an erection or vaginal lubrication–swelling?
3. Is your orgasm delayed or absent?
4. Do you experience premature ejaculation?
5. Do you have involuntary vaginal spasm during coitus?
6. Do you have pain during intercourse?

If sexual dysfunction is suspected, a more detailed sexual history may be indicated. The patient's previous experiences and his or her current beliefs and practices must be assessed. Pertinent information includes history of physical or sexual abuse, age at initial sexual contact, context of previous sexual contacts, history of abortion or miscarriage, reproductive history, and contraceptive history. An assessment of high-risk sexual activities must be made and a history of sexually transmitted diseases must be taken. Sexual problems often reflect some difficulty in a couple's relationship—for example, unstated or unconscious anger or frustration—so an understanding of the relationship may be helpful. A full assessment of sexual dysfunction includes a detailed medical, surgical, and pharmacological history. In addition, primary care practitioners will need to assess the patient for psychiatric symptoms. Sexual dysfunctions are highly prevalent among patients with mood disorders, anxiety disorders, psychosis, substance abuse disorders, and certain personality disorders.

Medication History

Many commonly used drugs interfere with sexual function. Antihypertensive and psychiatric drugs are common offenders. By informing patients of possible sexual side effects, practitioners will improve patient compliance and satisfaction.

Dysfunction that occurs with one antihypertensive may not occur with another. Thiazide diuretics, clonidine, and β-blockers have been implicated in impotence and loss of libido (10, 11). The angiotensin-converting enzyme inhibitors and the calcium channel blockers are less likely to produce sexual side effects (11). Other drugs cited as causing sexual dysfunction include cimetidine, antiandrogens, and antiestrogens (11).

Most antidepressants—including the serotonergic drugs, the tricyclic antidepressants, and the monoamine oxidase inhibitors—cause sexual dysfunction, including problems with libido, potency, and orgasm. Nefazodone and bupropion do not have the sexual side effects of other antidepressants. Trazodone can cause priapism and, along with bupropion, is thought to have prosexual effects. Most antipsychotic drugs raise prolactin levels, which may lead to decreased libido and impotence (10). In large studies, benzodiazepines have not been found to cause significant sexual dysfunction. However, case reports indicate problems with ejaculation and orgasm (11). At low dosages, benzodiazepines generally produce disinhibition and may enhance libido. At high dosages, sedation is produced. Drug-induced sexual dysfunction is usually dosage dependent and reversible.

Physical Examination

Most patients with sexual dysfunction will require a complete physical examination. Special attention should be paid to the neurological examination, the peripheral vascular examination, and the genitourinary examination. Table 8–2 lists pertinent parts of the physical examination (9).

Laboratory Testing

The laboratory workup should be guided by patient age, associated symptoms, and physical findings. Table 8–3 lists some recommended tests (9).

TABLE 8–2. **Physical examination to assess for sexual dysfunction**

Part of examination	What to look for
Skin	Signs of androgen activity (e.g., beard, balding, axillary hair), signs of alcohol abuse (e.g., palmar erythema)
Breasts	Men: gynecomastia as evidence of alcohol abuse or estrogen excess
	Men and women: galactorrhea may indicate a pituitary adenoma
External genitalia	Penis: size, shape, sensation, discharge, lesions, strictures
	Testes/scrotum: size, any evidence of atrophy, masses, tenderness, varicocele
	Clitoris, labia, vagina: size, sensation, lesions
Prostate	Size, nodules, tenderness
Rectum	Tone and lesions
Neurological system	Neuropathy
Peripheral vasculature	Pulses for evidence of vascular insufficiency

TABLE 8–3. **Recommended laboratory tests for evaluation of sexual dysfunction**

Hemoglobin and hematocrit
Liver function tests
Tests of renal function
Thyroid function tests
Workup for peripheral neuropathy: serum glucose, vitamin B_{12}, rapid plasma reagin test
For women:
  Serum estradiol
  Follicle-stimulating hormone, luteinizing hormone
  Androgen levels: testosterone, dehydroepiandrosterone sulfate
  Prolactin level
  Wet mount of vaginal secretions to diagnose vaginitis
For men:
  Testosterone level
  Prolactin level

■ SPECIFIC DISORDERS AND TREATMENT

Treatment involves a variety of modalities. Because some patients are unwilling to see psychiatrists or sex therapists, primary care practitioners may need to provide counseling and education to patients and their partners. Referral to relevant literature available to the general public is helpful.

A plethora of psychological techniques are available for treating sexual disorders. For these techniques to be successful, however, referral to a specialist often is necessary. Community counseling centers may be a useful resource for referrals to sex therapists.

Sexual Desire Disorders

Disorders of sexual desire range from a paucity of fantasy and desire (hypoactive sexual desire disorder) to an absolute aversion to most or all sexual contact (sexual aversion disorder) to an uncontrollable desire to seek sexual gratification (so-called sex addiction). The dysfunction, no matter what its form, must cause marked difficulty for the patient before the diagnosis can be made. In making the diagnosis, the practitioner must also ascertain whether the lack of desire is specific to a particular situation or partner or whether it is a general deficiency in sexual interests. The latter is more suggestive of a genuine dysfunction and not simply a relationship or situational problem.

Hypoactive sexual desire disorder. Hypoactive sexual desire disorder is thought to be common in both men and women (1) and can have both medical and psychological causes. Common organic problems associated with loss of desire include chronic illnesses, such as diabetes and multiple sclerosis, and certain hormonal changes, such as pregnancy, menopause, or lower-than-normal circulating testosterone levels. Alcohol and drugs can also cause decreased desire in men and women who consume them regularly (12). Psychological factors that can lead to lack of desire include chronic stress, depression, anxiety, poor self-esteem, and marital strife.

This disorder is one of the most difficult sexual dysfunctions to treat. Replacement estrogens and androgens restore sexual function only in those with clinical hypogonadism or other hormonal abnormalities (13). Testosterone has been used with equivocal results, and in women, the masculinizing effects are a problem. Yohimbine, an α_2-adrenoceptor antagonist, has been shown to increase libido (13). Other described treatments involve the use of specialized forms of psychotherapy such as marital therapy to improve communication within the couple, cognitive-behavioral therapy to address distorted beliefs about sex, modified Masters and Johnson's sex therapy, and behavioral exercises that increase sexual pleasure and decrease anxiety.

Sexual aversion disorder. Sexual aversion disorder is a severe form of sexual desire disorder that is sometimes referred to as *sexual phobia.* The individual reports anxiety, fear, or disgust when confronted by a sexual opportunity with a partner, and he or she actively avoids genital sexual contact (14). Aversion to sexual activity may result from a traumatic sexual experience, repeated painful sexual activity, or early childhood conflicts that cause excessive shame and guilt (15). Systematic desensitization can reduce anxiety. Tricyclic antidepressants have been reported to help (15).

Sex addiction. Sex addiction is not a recognized nosological term, but it has been described in the literature. It is not to be confused with addictions seen in patients who are substance dependent, wherein physiological and psychological changes occur as a result of chronic use of the substance. Sex addiction is characterized by excessive amounts of time spent planning and engaging in sexual activities. In many patients, the disorder is comorbid with other psychiatric disorders and substance abuse. Management is primarily through self-help groups based on the 12-step Alcoholics Anonymous model. Other therapies that require the assistance of mental health specialists include insight-oriented therapy, which facilitates an understanding of the causes of the behavior, and cognitive-behavioral therapy. Medications such as serotonin reuptake inhibitors, medroxyprogesterone acetate, and antiandrogens may help decrease the sex drive, although no large systematic studies are available regarding their safety and efficacy (15).

Sexual Arousal Disorders

Arousal disorder in women. Arousal disorder in women involves a persistent inability to attain or maintain a lubrication-swelling response until the sexual activity is completed. The definition emphasizes the absence of physiological arousal, even though lack of subjective arousal is usually the suspected cause (16). The disorder may lead to painful intercourse, but the disorder may be masked in many women who use vaginal lubricants (16). Physical conditions such as systemic illnesses should be ruled out.

Common endocrinological factors leading to decreased lubrication and arousal include alteration of hormones such as testosterone, estrogen, prolactin, and thyroxine (15). Postmenopausal women, especially, may need more time to achieve adequate vaginal lubrication. Furthermore, medications such as anticholinergic and antihistaminic agents may adversely affect lubrication and arousal. A solitary diagnosis of female sexual arousal disorder independent of orgasmic or desire disorders is unlikely (16).

Various treatment strategies have been recommended, including the use of artificial lubricants, estrogen replacement therapy (for postmenopausal women), sex therapy, couples therapy, and fantasy training. Other techniques include sensate focus procedures, graduated directed self-stimulation, interventions to increase generalized autonomic arousal (e.g., exercise), and biofeedback. Kegel exercises, primarily used for treating urinary incontinence, strengthen the pubococcygeal muscle, which reportedly helps increase sexual arousal. No oral pharmacological agents are helpful in treating this condition.

Male erectile disorder. This disorder, more commonly known as *impotence,* is the most prevalent sexual disorder of men seen in sex therapy clinics (16). The condition is characterized by an inability to achieve and maintain an erection until the completion of a sexual act. Common organic causes include diabetes (the most common); chronic cardiovascular and neurological disorders; pituitary, adrenal, and thyroid disorders; hematologic, hepatic, pulmonary, and renal disorders; and pelvic surgery, trauma, or infection. The occurrence of spontaneous erections, particularly in the morning, and the ability to masturbate lessen the probability of an organic etiology. The presence of a medical condition that may cause impotence does not rule out psychological factors as the primary reason for the dysfunction.

Psychological factors implicated in erectile dysfunction include fear, feelings of shame and guilt, so-called performance anxiety, and unresolved conflicts with a partner. Assuring the patient that most men have had periods of impotence can alleviate anxiety, which worsens the dysfunction. Behavioral strategies and psychological treatments have been successful, but biological treatments have been developed more recently. These treatments include intracavernous injections; use of oral pharmacological agents, surgical prostheses, external vacuum devices, and constriction rings; and vascular surgeries. If a vascular problem is suspected, Doppler examination should be used to check penile blood flow.

Intracavernous injections are commonly used in urological clinics. Intracavernous prostaglandin E1 injection is most often preferred because of a lower incidence of side effects, but intraurethral prostaglandins have been used recently. Prostaglandin E1 is a potent smooth-muscle relaxant and vasodilator in humans (17). Dosing does not have to be altered in patients who have hepatic or renal insufficiency (17). Intracavernous prostaglandin E1 is effective for erectile dysfunction of neurogenic, vasculogenic, psychogenic, and mixed origin; however, neither prostaglandin E1 nor sildenafil (see below) is effective in men with severe arterial insufficiency, loss of trabecular smooth muscle or incompressible cavernosal veins (18). The use of prostaglandin E1 is contraindicated in patients who have sickle cell anemia or trait, multiple myeloma, leukemia, or preexisting corporal fibrosis or tunica plaques, which can complicate frequent intracavernous injections (17). Titration of the dosage should be done in a physician's office by trained personnel, and the optimal recommended duration of erection is 1 hour.

Oral pharmacological agents hold considerable promise for the treatment of erectile disorder. Yohimbine increases penile blood inflow and restricts penile venous outflow. It has been used for psychogenic and biological erectile disorders. The recommended dosage is 5.4 mg three times a day. Studies of its efficacy have had mixed results.

With sexual stimulation, nitrous oxide is released in the corpora cavernosa, which induces the formation of cyclic guanosine monophosphate (GMP). Cyclic GMP acts to relax arterial smooth muscle so that blood flow increases in the penis and erection ensues (19). Sildenafil (Viagra) inhibits the breakdown of cyclic GMP and is effective in treating impotence in patients with diabetes, those with spinal cord injuries, those who have had a prostatectomy, and those taking antidepressants (although it has not been studied with the selective serotonin reuptake inhibitors) and/or antipsychotics (18). Unlike prostaglandin E1, sildenafil is only effective if accompanied by sexual stimulation (19). Men without erectile disorder report that sildenafil helps with achieving and maintaining an erection (18). It has not been studied in women as of this writing.

The manufacturer recommends an initial dose of 50 mg 1 hour prior to sexual intercourse, although it can be taken from ½ hour to 4 hours before intercourse. The maximum dose is 100 mg daily, but lower dosages should be used in the elderly and those with hepatic or renal disease (18). Patients need to be told not to take any compounds containing nitrates, such as sublingual nitroglycerin or amyl nitrate (which is used as an aphrodisiac), simultaneously with sildenafil, because the combination can result in marked hypotension (18). Although sildenafil will prove to be helpful to many men, practitioners are still advised to do a thorough evaluation before prescribing sildenafil and will need guidelines concerning its use in men without impotence (19).

Nonresponse to pharmacological measures may be an indication for the use of penile prostheses. Several types of prostheses are available, and referral should be made to a urologist to determine which device is indicated for the patient. A noninvasive alternative to penile implants is external vacuum devices, which can be helpful for impotence caused by psychological factors, mild vascular insufficiency, and neurogenic disorders.

Orgasmic Disorders

Female orgasmic disorder. Female orgasmic disorder involves a persistent and frequent delay in orgasm, or the inability to reach orgasm, following a normal sexual excitement phase. It may be classified as either lifelong (primary) or acquired (secondary). The former type has a better prognosis than the latter. The practitioner must consider the patient's previous sexual experience when making the diagnosis because increased orgasmic potential is expected in more experienced individuals. The practitioner must rule out organic causes, such as endocrinological disorders (e.g., diabetes, hypothyroidism, hyperprolactinemia) and medications (e.g., antihypertensives and antidepressants). Psychological causes include obsessive self-observation during sex, unresolved marital conflict, inability to abandon oneself to pleasure, and insufficient stimulation for orgasm (15). Societal norms and strong religious beliefs may also play a significant role in orgasmic inhibition. For women who have general anorgasmia, sex therapy and directed self-stimulation exercises may be warranted. Informing the patient that not all intercourse leads to female orgasm may ease the inhibition. In situations in which the anorgasmia is situational, treatment outcome is less positive. The disorder is often associated with psychiatric disorders or relationship conflicts and thus warrants appropriate referral. Pharmacological interventions have yet to be developed.

Male orgasmic disorder. Male orgasmic disorder usually involves inhibited male orgasm or retarded ejaculation. It is a persistent or frequent delay in, or the absence of, orgasm following a normal sexual excitement phase. The prevalence of this condition is quite low relative to premature ejaculation and male erectile disorder, although a higher prevalence has been reported among homosexual men (16). This disorder must be differentiated from retrograde ejaculation, in which orgasm and ejaculation occur but the semen is shunted to the bladder. Retrograde ejaculation is usually the result of organic causes such as genitourinary procedures or medications with anticholinergic properties. Biological causes of male orgasmic disorder include Parkinson's disease and spinal cord lesions. Antihypertensives, antidepressants, antipsychotics, and excessive alcohol intake may also produce this condition. Psychological and interpersonal factors have been implicated in the development of the disorder. These factors include performance anxiety, fear of impregnating the partner, lack of desire or arousal, or conflicted attitudes about sex (15). Male orgasmic disorder is more difficult to treat than is female orgasmic disorder, and referral should be made to a mental health professional after biological causes are ruled out.

Premature ejaculation. This disorder involves a persistent or frequent ejaculation with minimal stimulation before, during, or immediately after penetration and before the person wishes it. The clinician must consider the patient's age, sexual experience, and frequency of sexual activity in making the diagnosis. Organic conditions are rarely implicated, but surgical trauma, pelvic fracture, local genital disease, and withdrawal from narcotics have been associated with premature ejaculation. Premature ejaculation is commonly associated with high levels of anxiety and arousal. Ongoing stress in a relationship may also cause this condition. Treatment approaches for premature ejaculation include the traditional pause-and-squeeze techniques developed by Semans and Masters and Johnson and cognitive-behavioral interventions.

Pharmacological agents have been helpful in the treatment of premature ejaculation. Twenty-five milligrams of amitriptyline may be taken 3–5 hours prior to intercourse. Phenoxybenzamine, an α-adrenergic antagonist, at 20–30 mg/day is also used. Low-dose clomipramine (25 and 50 mg) can significantly lengthen ejaculatory latencies (20, 21). Recent reports have also documented the efficacy of low-dose serotonergic agents (e.g., fluoxetine and sertraline) in premature ejaculation.

Pain Disorders

Dyspareunia, or painful intercourse, is a highly prevalent disorder in women, but it is relatively rare in men. It is the most common sexual complaint spontaneously reported to gynecologists. In women, physical factors are important. Specific causes of dyspareunia include infections such as pelvic inflammatory disease, herpes simplex, and candidal infection; vulvar vestibulitis (a recently described condition); endometriosis; scarring of the hymen and vaginal stenosis; allergic reactions to deodorants or contraceptive materials; vaginismus; and gastrointestinal disease such as hemorrhoids, constipation, and proctitis.

Vulvar vestibulitis is characterized by pain at the introitus and, often, erythema. The etiology is unknown, and histological examination shows evidence of mild to moderate inflammation in the epithelium (22). A gynecologist is best qualified to make the diagnosis, although there is no consensus on treatment (23).

Essential vulvodynia, or dysesthetic vulvodynia, is most common among women who are perimenopausal or postmenopausal (22). There are no significant findings on physical examination, and the pain is similar to that of postherpetic neuralgia (22). Tricyclic antidepressants may improve symptoms. Vulvar pain, like other pain syndromes, provokes psychological distress and may make a woman feel less desirable. This distress may precipitate problems with spousal or other significant relationships. Counseling is an important aspect of management.

Vaginismus is characterized by involuntary spasms in the muscles of the outer third of the vagina and is seen relatively often in sex therapy clinics. *Primary vaginismus* refers to involuntary vaginal spasm that occurs in all situations, so that patients even avoid gynecological examinations. *Secondary vaginismus* refers to a condition in which some penetration is possible. Psychological factors associated with vaginismus are a history of sexual trauma and conflicts about sexual issues (16).

Treatment approaches for female dyspareunia include the appropriate medical or surgical interventions for the specific pathology. Estrogen replacement therapy may help alleviate vaginal dryness and postcoital bleeding in postmenopausal women. Transdermal estrogen may be the preferred route of administration because it avoids first-pass metabolic effects on the liver. In addition, most women will require adjunctive cognitive-behavioral or sex therapy in order to have intercourse successfully and to ameliorate the problems of anxiety and lack of arousal (16). Treatment of vaginismus will generally combine the use of vaginal dilators with systematic desensitization and pubococcygeal muscle training (16).

Sexual Disorders in Selected Populations

Geriatric patients. Sexual activity in the aged population is influenced strongly by the availability of a partner and the individual's health status. Biological factors and medications are likely to play a role in newly acquired sexual dysfunction at this age. However, sexual feelings are as important in this age group as in any other. Touching and caressing without intercourse is the most common sexual activity for both men and women (24). Dyspareunia is a common sexual complaint of women seeking medical consultation for sexual problems and often results from thinning of the vaginal walls and a decrease in vaginal secretions. Orgasmic response is not impaired significantly in older women (25). Men do not experience the dramatic change in sex hormones with aging that occurs in women. The decrease in testosterone levels is gradual in aging men. Little evidence indicates that testosterone replacement will significantly improve sexual function in older men who have testosterone levels within the normal range (25). Erectile difficulty is the most common sexual complaint of older men (25).

Patients with medical conditions. Medical conditions, such as a recent myocardial infarction, may provide a psychological impediment to sexual activity, but patients should be advised that they can safely resume sexual activity. Clinicians should specifically discuss sexual activity after an illness. Sexual activity may need to be modified for patients with certain disabilities. If arthritic pain is a problem, pain medication timed carefully before intercourse may help. In older patients, the side-to-side position may be preferable to having one partner lying on top of the other. Sensual alternatives to genital sex can be discussed.

Homosexual patients. A homosexual orientation is not considered a clinical problem unless it is distressing to the individual. Because there is significant societal prejudice against homosexuals, eliciting an accurate relationship and sexual history may be difficult. Human immunodeficiency virus (HIV) infection risk is a consideration among homosexual men. The adoption of safe sex practices among the homosexual male population is far from universal, although this population is more likely to have adopted safe sex practices than the analogous heterosexual population. The majority of lesbian women begin same-gender sexual activity after age 18 (26). Most homosexuals are hesitant to discuss their sexual orientation with practitioners whom they perceive to be hostile to their sexual practices.

■ CONCLUSION

Sexuality is a highly personal area of function for men and women. Some areas of sexual dysfunction are amenable to treatment, such as premature ejaculation and erectile disorders in men, whereas in other disorders, such as inhibited orgasm, the pathophysiology is little understood and effective treatments are lacking. Because sexual dysfunction can be embarrassing, a sensitive discussion will take time and interest on the part of the practitioner. Routine screening instruments for sexual dysfunction have not gained acceptance in primary care nor can one particular instrument be recommended at this time. Practitioners who demonstrate an openness to discussion and to the treatment possibilities in this area will be rewarded with improved patient satisfaction.

■ REFERENCES

1. Halvorsen JG, Metz ME: Sexual dysfunction, part 1: classification, etiology, and pathogenesis. J Am Board Fam Pract 5:51–61, 1992
2. Rushton DN: Sexual and sphincter dysfunction, in Neurology in Clinical Practice. Edited by Bradley WG. Boston, MA, Butterworth-Heinemann, 1996, pp 415–420
3. Spector IP, Carey MP: Incidence and prevalence of the sexual dysfunctions: a critical review of the empirical literature. Arch Sex Behav 19:384–408, 1990

4. Miccoli R, Giampetro O, Tognarelli M, et al: Prevalence and types of sexual dysfunctions in diabetic males: a standardized and clinical approach. J Med 18:305–321, 1987
5. Monga TN, Lawson JS, Inglis J: Sexual dysfunction in stroke patients. Arch Phys Med Rehabil 67:19–22, 1986
6. Tardif GS: Sexual activity after a myocardial infarction. Arch Phys Med Rehabil 70:763–766, 1989
7. Mattson D, Petrie M, Srivastava DK, et al: Multiple sclerosis: sexual dysfunction and its response to medications. Arch Neurol 52:862–868, 1995
8. Driscoll CE, Garner EG, House JD: The effect of taking a sexual history on the notation of sexually related diagnoses. Fam Med 18:293–295, 1986
9. Kligman EW: Office evaluation of sexual function and complaints. Clin Geriatr Med 7:15–39, 1991
10. Abramowicz ME: Drugs that cause sexual dysfunction: an update. Med Lett Drugs Ther 34:73–76, 1991
11. Deamer R, Thompson J: The role of medications in geriatric sexual function. Clin Geriatr Med 7:95–111, 1991
12. Miller NS, Gold MS: The human sexual response and alcohol and drugs. J Subst Abuse Treat 5:171–177, 1988
13. Rosen RC, Ashton AK: Prosexual drugs: empirical status of the "new aphrodisiacs." Arch Sex Behav 22:521–543, 1993
14. American Psychiatric Association: Diagnostic and Statistical Manual of Mental Disorders, 4th Edition. Washington, DC, American Psychiatric Association, 1994
15. Sadock VA: Normal human sexuality and sexual and gender identity disorders, in Comprehensive Textbook of Psychiatry, 6th Edition. Edited by Kaplan HI, Sadock BJ. Baltimore, MD, Williams & Wilkins, 1995, pp 1295–1321
16. Rosen R, Leiblum S: Treatment of sexual disorders in the 1990s: an integrated approach. J Consult Clin Psychol 63:877–890, 1995
17. Broderick GA: Intracavernous pharmacotherapy. Urol Clin North Am 23:111–126, 1996
18. Gelenberg AJ: Sildenafil (Viagra). Biological Therapies in Psychiatry Newsletter 21:25–26, 1998
19. Utiger RD: A pill for impotence. N Engl J Med 338:1458–1459, 1998
20. Segraves RT, Saran A, Segraves K, et al: Clomipramine versus placebo in the treatment of premature ejaculation: a pilot study. J Sex Marital Ther 19:198–200, 1993

21. Althof SE, Levine SB, Corty EW, et al: A double blind cross-over trial of clomipramine for rapid ejaculation in 15 couples. J Clin Psychiatry 56:402–407, 1995
22. Paavonen J: Diagnosis and treatment of vulvodynia. Ann Med 27: 175–181, 1995
23. Baggish MS: Vulvar pain syndrome: a review. Obstet Gynecol Surv 50:618–627, 1995
24. Bretschneider J, McCoy N: Sexual interest and behavior in healthy 80- to 102-year-olds. Arch Sex Behav 17:109–130, 1988
25. Leiblum S, Segraves R: Sex and aging, in American Psychiatric Press Review of Psychiatry, Vol 14. Edited by Oldham JM, Riba MB. Washington, DC, American Psychiatric Press, 1995, pp 677–695
26. Seidman SN, Rieder RO: Sexual behavior through the life cycle: an empirical approach, in American Psychiatric Press Review of Psychiatry, Vol 14. Edited by Oldham JM, Riba MB. Washington, DC, American Psychiatric Press, 1995, pp 639–676

9

SLEEP DISORDERS

Joyce R. Zinsenheim, M.D.

Sleep is a natural, periodic, and reversible state that changes in quantity and quality throughout the life cycle. Newborn infants sleep approximately 17 hours daily and lack diurnal rhythmicity. By 6 months of age, a child's sleep is consolidated into 8- to 12-hour nocturnal sleep periods with two to four naps ranging in length from 1 to 4 hours. The sleep period normally attains nocturnal predominance with a gradual diminution of naps through the preschool years. There continues to be a diminution in total sleep time from 11 hours at age 5 to 8¼ hours at age 17. There are further changes in sleep that occur as people age, as will be discussed below.

There are two types of sleep: non–rapid eye movement (NREM) and rapid eye movement (REM). NREM sleep has four stages. In stages 1 and 2, sleep is light. Stages 3 and 4 are called deep, delta, or slow-wave sleep. Delta sleep predominates in the first half of the night, and it diminishes with age. Sleep is entered via stage 1, which is a brief transitional stage; if awakened during stage 1, a patient will report that he or she has not been asleep. Stage 2 is slightly deeper than stage 1 and accounts for 50% of adult sleep. Stages 3 and 4 occupy 10%–20% of net sleep time (1).

REM sleep is normally entered after approximately 90 minutes of NREM sleep and is characterized by the paradoxical features of muscle atony in the presence of low-amplitude, mixed-frequency electroencephalographic waves, and rapid eye movements. It accounts for 20%–25% of adult sleep and occurs in four to six distinct periods (1). It tends to predominate in the second half of the sleep period. Dream activity is limited largely to REM sleep.

NREM and REM sleep occur in a cyclical pattern but may be punctuated by either internal stimuli (e.g., the need to urinate) or external stimuli (e.g., noise). The occurrence and stability of the sleep cycles and stages can also be altered by many medical and psychiatric conditions, by the use of drugs and alcohol, and by altered sleep-wake-work patterns.

Sleep efficiency (sleep time measured as a percentage of total time in bed) begins to decline after age 45 (2). Other changes in sleep that occur as people age include fragmentation (i.e., the patient experiences more awakenings during the night and has more difficulty falling back asleep), less slow-wave sleep, and more sleep in NREM stage 1 (2).

■ EVALUATION

Sleep disturbances are generally symptomatic of other underlying conditions and should be addressed through a comprehensive evaluation. The sleep history should include current and past sleep habits, drug and alcohol use, and medical and psychiatric history. The symptoms should be corroborated by a bed partner, if available. A diary of sleep and wake times is helpful in the assessment.

Sleep disturbances are best approached using the inventory shown in Table 9–1. The inventory should be followed by a physical examination.

■ SPECIFIC DISORDERS

Table 9–2 summarizes the essential clinical features of the sleep disorders and their treatment.

Psychophysiological Insomnia

Chronic psychophysiological insomnia is considered to be a learned behavioral condition associated with complaints of cognitive dysfunction, reduced energy, and nonspecific somatic symp-

TABLE 9–1. **Sleep inventory**

Typical bedtime and awakening times
Time spent awake in bed
Frequency and duration of awakenings
Presence of snoring, gasping, or leg movements
Daytime alertness
Use of alcohol, medications (including over-the-counter), and caffeine
Assessment of psychiatric disorders
Sleep environment
Eating habits at bedtime
Former sleep patterns

toms. The condition usually begins with a stressor and several successive nights of poor-quality, nonrestorative sleep. Maladaptive techniques such as "trying hard" to sleep exacerbate the insomnia. To compensate for the loss of sleep, patients may take naps. The fragmentation of sleep and preoccupation with falling asleep enter a cyclical phase that is difficult to address and correct without careful review. A brief trial of sedative-hypnotics and maintenance of sleep hygiene (discussed later in this chapter [also refer to Table 9–3, below]) are the mainstays of treatment.

Narcolepsy

Narcolepsy is a condition of abnormal REM activity associated with hypersomnolence. It may appear insidiously in adolescence but it is not usually recognized until 10–15 years later, when the individual's school or job performance becomes impaired. Narcolepsy is associated with four distinctive clinical symptoms:

1. Excessive daytime sleepiness
2. Sleep paralysis
3. Hypnagogic (on falling asleep) and hypnopompic (on awakening) hallucinations
4. Cataplexy (loss of muscle tone)

TABLE 9–2. **Clinical features of the sleep disorders and their treatment**

Disorder	Clinical feature(s)	Treatment
Psychophysiological insomnia	Preceded by stressor(s)	Sleep hygiene
	Nonrestorative sleep	Brief trial of hypnotics
Narcolepsy	Sleep attacks	Psychostimulants
	Cataplexy	Tricyclic antidepressants
Obstructive sleep apnea	Airflow obstruction during sleep	Continuous positive airway pressure
	Snoring	Avoidance of benzodiazepines
	Restless sleep	Protriptyline
	Daytime drowsiness	Surgery
Primary snoring; upper airway resistance syndrome	Similar to obstructive sleep apnea but no oxyhemoglobin desaturations	Avoidance of sleeping in supine position
Periodic limb movements	Involuntary movement of extremities	Clonazepam
		L-dopa/carbidopa
Restless legs syndrome	Cramps or aches in lower extremities	Same as periodic limb movements
Substance-related sleep disorder	Substance causes sleep disruption	Discontinuation of substance
Circadian rhythm disorder	Sleep-wake cycle altered by travel, work, or habit	Brief trial of hypnotics
		Chronotherapy
		Phototherapy
Parasomnias	Partial awakening and unusual behaviors	Benzodiazepines for REM disorder

Sleep attacks may occur when the patient feels bored, and cataplexy can be induced when the patient experiences strong emotions such as fear (3). Narcolepsy is diagnosed with polysomnography, which is conducted at sleep disorder centers. In patients with narcolepsy, REM sleep occurs during daytime hours, and the REM latency time (the time it takes to enter REM sleep) is less than 5 minutes (4). Patients with narcolepsy should be referred to a specialist for initiation of treatment. Pharmacotherapy includes the use of psychostimulants such as methylphenidate. The tricyclic antidepressants are used to treat cataplexy.

Obstructive Sleep Apnea

Apnea is defined as the cessation of breathing through the nose and mouth for 10 seconds or more (5). Three types of apnea exist. Central apnea is not common and occurs when respiratory movements of the thorax and abdomen are lacking. In obstructive sleep apnea (OSA), airflow is blocked in the upper airway such that 50%–60% of total sleep time is without adequate airflow (2). Mixed apnea occurs when the absent muscle movement is followed by airway obstruction. All three types may be observed in the same patient (3).

OSA is more prevalent in older men (5, 6) and may be associated with obesity and hypertension (5). It is characterized by four chief symptoms:

1. Loud and irregular snoring
2. Breathing pauses
3. Restless sleep
4. Daytime drowsiness

Patients sometimes misinterpret their symptoms and perceive that they have insomnia. This misinterpretation can occur especially if the individual sleeps alone and is unaware of the gasping and irregular breathing that accompany apneic episodes. The events may terminate with a partial awakening and position change. The patient then returns to sleep briefly, and multiple episodes recur throughout the night.

Obstructive respiratory events may range from total obstruction (apnea) of the airway to partial obstruction (hypopnea) and may be associated with quiet to very loud snoring. During apneic periods, arterial oxygen desaturations of under 85% may occur (2). Sleep apnea patients may develop pulmonary hypertension, polycythemia, and cardiac dysrhythmias. Some alterations of blood pressure, blood flow, skin temperature, and respirations are normal in REM sleep; however, these changes can be severely exaggerated in patients with OSA.

Individuals may complain of fatigue, memory loss, mood changes, and insomnia. These symptoms may be misinterpreted as indicating major depression. Clinical features on physical examination include upper airway abnormalities such as retrognathism, tonsillar and uvular hypertrophy, large neck diameter (in excess of 17 inches), hypertension, increased abdominal girth, and, in more severe cases, signs of congestive heart failure. Any individual who exhibits these features and has a history of loud snoring and fatigue should be referred for prompt testing with polysomnography.

Treatment of OSA begins with a positive pressure delivery system such as nasal continuous positive airway pressure (CPAP). CPAP and related positive pressure devices require nightly use of the device to maintain airway patency during sleep. CPAP is highly effective despite a high discontinuation rate. It remains the standard for treatment of OSA. Patients also should be encouraged to lose weight, if appropriate (7); restrict alcohol intake (8), especially within 4 hours of bedtime; and, in most cases, avoid myorelaxant agents such as benzodiazepines (9).

Primary snoring and a relatively newly described clinical syndrome, upper airway resistance syndrome (UARS), are frequently overlooked by clinicians evaluating patients who complain of insomnia and daytime hypersomnolence. Both conditions are characterized by fragmented sleep and an absence of oxyhemoglobin desaturations. Paradoxical breathing (desynchronized chest and abdominal movement) is observed in both OSA and UARS. Position therapy (i.e., avoidance of the supine sleep position) is encouraged, to reduce sleep fragmentation. This therapy may be performed by placing two tennis balls into a back pajama pocket, which prevents the individual from sleeping in the supine position (10).

Pharmacological treatment continues to be a rather limited option. Studies have demonstrated some improvement in patients with mild to moderate sleep apnea with protriptyline, an activating tricyclic antidepressant (11, 12). The anticholinergic effects of dry mouth, constipation, urinary retention, confusion, and ataxia have tempered the enthusiasm for pharmacotherapy with tricyclic antidepressants. Protriptyline is not indicated for severe OSA.

Surgical options for OSA and snoring have become more refined, but they have inconsistent outcomes. Surgical procedures vary from the newer and popular outpatient procedures such as laser-assisted uvulopalatoplasty (LAUP) to septoplasty, uvulopalatoplasty (UPP), mandibular advancement, and tracheostomy. LAUP is seen as an attractive alternative for many patients who cannot or will not use the CPAP device, and it is indicated in patients with primary snoring, UARS, or mild OSA. Additional studies are needed before unequivocal support for these procedures can be given.

Dental appliances also have a respectable following but are less enthusiastically endorsed for most OSA patients because of the limited number of peer-reviewed studies of these devices. These devices protect the airway either by retaining the tongue away from the posterior airway space or by repositioning the mandible. An oral appliance may be helpful for mild sleep apnea but should not be recommended for severe sleep apnea.

Periodic Limb Movements and Restless Legs Syndrome

Many patients complain of fragmented sleep and increased body movements. Periodic limb movements (PLMs) are characterized by sudden, involuntary extremity movements occurring during sleep. They are more common in the elderly (13). Partial or full awakenings can cause confusion at the time of the event or fatigue and drowsiness during the following day. Patients may exacerbate the problem by self-medicating with alcohol or over-the-counter agents to promote consolidation of sleep. Upper—or, more commonly, lower—extremity movements occur approximately every 20–40 seconds, usually in clusters. The clusters may last a few minutes to hours. The classical movements resemble the Babinski reflex. The great toe extends with simultaneous flexion of the toes, ankle, and leg, and occasionally flexion of the hip and knee. A bed partner may observe these quick leg movements but more commonly reports the patient as restless. The patient may deny disturbances, with only vague complaints of mood changes, irritability, impaired memory, decreased concentration, and poor job performance.

Restless legs syndrome (RLS) is less common than are PLMs. RLS patients typically describe cramping, aching, or tingling sensations of the lower extremities, which are relieved with vigorous leg movement or massage. These frequently painful sensations are usually idiopathic and may begin in childhood. Patients may "walk the floors," jump, or perform elaborate leg movements to extinguish the sensations, which are worst during inactivity, especially at bedtime. Patients frequently present to clinicians highly distressed with complaints of chronic insomnia and jumpiness and a history of self-medication to control the movements and to promote sleep. RLS can be mistaken for and misdiagnosed as the more common anxiety disorders because of the intense and distracting motor activity. Many patients state they are sleepy until they go to bed, when kicking and movement urgency occurs.

These two sleep disorders are commonly overlooked by patients and practitioners. Careful historical evaluation with polysomnography can confirm the diagnosis of PLMs, whereas RLS can usually be diagnosed by history. Treatment consists of administration of benzodiazepines, which do not fully block the movements but suppress the arousals generated by the movements. Clonazepam (Klonopin) and temazepam (Restoril) have been used with favorable results (14). Many specialists prefer to use the dopaminergic agents such as L-dopa/carbidopa to suppress the leg movements. Rebound leg movements can occur. Other dopaminergic agonists, such as bromocriptine (Parlodel) and pergolide (Permax), have been used successfully, and baclofen, opiates, carbamazepine, and adrenergic agents have also been effective. Newer anticonvulsant agents such as gabapentin have been useful for treating highly refractory disorders (15). Treatment with these agents should be initiated by a sleep specialist.

Substance-Dependent Sleep Disorders

Sleep disorders can arise because of the use of substances. For example, patients can become tolerant to the hypnotic benzodiazepines and take higher dosages to help them sleep, leading to a new level of tolerance and insomnia; thus, the cycle repeats itself. Patients who are dependent on hypnotics should undergo a gradual detoxification.

Stimulant-dependent sleep disorder can arise from the misuse of xanthine-containing beverages, such as coffee, tea, and hot chocolate, and other caffeinated agents. Caffeine increases wakefulness and reduces delta sleep and total sleep time. Many over-the-counter agents contain caffeine, and not all product labels clearly indicate the quantity of caffeine in each tablet. Amphetamines and their related heterocyclic derivatives and over-the-counter diet pills increase wakefulness. Sleep onset can be delayed and sleep continuity disrupted with acute or chronic stimulant use. Many patients require no other management than discontinuation of all caffeinated substances. Caffeine should be withdrawn gradually.

Alcohol can appear to be an ideal hypnotic agent because it is readily available, requires no prescription, and is initially quite successful in inducing sleep. *Sleep latency,* the time it takes to fall asleep, is abbreviated with a small amount of alcohol, which suppresses wakefulness for approximately 4 hours, at which point the alcohol is metabolized. Alcohol is thus effective for individuals who have initial and middle insomnia. Sleep may feel more refreshing because alcohol may increase restorative delta sleep and suppresses REM. Once the alcohol level decreases, rebound insomnia symptoms appear with sleep fragmentation and, occasionally, REM rebound and diminished delta sleep. The REM rebound may cause very disturbing nightmares and wakefulness. Another dose of alcohol may help the patient to return to sleep, but over time, tolerance develops, with larger doses needed for the maintenance of increasingly shorter periods of sleep. Withdrawal and abstinence may cause prolonged periods of wakefulness lasting up to several days to weeks.

Circadian Rhythm Sleep Disorder

Time zone change syndrome is a circadian rhythm disturbance commonly known as *jet lag.* It occurs when the body's biological clock mismatches the surrounding environment. West-to-east travel is more troublesome than east-to-west travel for most people, owing to the inherent slightly phase-delayed circadian rhythm. The human body can adapt at the rate of one time zone per day. Many popular books offer both helpful and harmful suggestions. Patients should be encouraged to practice good sleep hygiene (described later in this chapter) prior to trip departure and to maintain the regular home schedule for short trips. Very short trips or multiple time zone changes may necessitate the use of a hypnotic for a short period. The benzodiazepine agents, such as temazepam, clonazepam, and lorazepam, can be used effectively in small doses. Zolpidem is also effective.

In delayed sleep phase syndrome, patients alter their sleep time to such an extent that they cannot adapt their sleep-wake cycle to conventional hours (e.g., those who work shifts or stay up late into the night). Under the direction of a specialist, the treatment (called chronotherapy) gradually reestablishes a regular sleep cycle.

Advanced sleep phase syndrome is commonly seen in the elderly and may begin insidiously. Boredom, arthritis, and pain from other medical conditions may promote early bedtime, thus advancing sleep time as early as 5:00 P.M. or 6:00 P.M. The normal sleep period may end approximately 6–7 hours later in the middle of the night. Corrective measures that promote wakefulness through activity may quickly terminate the process. Patients should be advised to avoid bed and reclining on the sofa until at least 9:00 P.M. They should not begin bedtime preparation, such as changing into pajamas, until they are ready to go to bed.

Delayed sleep phase syndrome and advanced sleep phase syndrome frequently respond to manipulation of the sleep-wake schedule, and pharmacological treatment should not be instituted until an adequate behavioral trial has failed. In phototherapy, another treatment method used by sleep specialists, the patient is exposed to bright fluorescent lights to reset the suprachiasmatic nucleus, the brain's pacemaker.

Parasomnias

Parasomnias are events that occur either in a sleep stage or immediately following a stimulus that causes partial awakening that allows for unusual behaviors. The most common examples are sleepwalking and sleep terrors. Sleepwalking occurs usually in children and occurs during the first third of the night's sleep. Pavor nocturnus (sleep terrors) are NREM behaviors that occur in sleep stages 3 and 4 and are seen most frequently in young children. Unlike nightmares, their hallmark features are sudden screams and uncontrollable crying and sobbing in an activated, inconsolable child. Sympathetic hyperactivity is demonstrated. The event terminates after several minutes, and most children do not remember the event. Medications are not indicated, and parents should be encouraged to protect the child but never to try to interrupt the state with loud noises, threats, or harsh treatment. These events are not psychiatric conditions but reflect a temporary dysregulation of sleep.

Nightmares can be distinguished from the parasomnias by the vivid dream content with prompt awakening and recall of the threatening and frightening themes. Nightmares, unlike night terrors, arise from REM sleep rather than from NREM sleep and may occur at any age. Many drugs can cause nightmares, owing to REM-activating properties.

REM behavior disorder is a fairly recently described disorder. The behaviors exhibited can appear complex, violent, and purposeful but are pathological because they occur in REM sleep, when motor activity should be limited to only eye movements and essential functions such as cardiac and respiratory activity. Diagnosis is made using polysomnography, and treatment is directed at suppressing REM sleep using benzodiazepines such as clonazepam.

Sleep Disorders Associated With a Psychiatric Disorder

Many psychiatric disorders affect sleep. Major depression is associated with a prolonged sleep latency, a shortened REM latency, early morning awakening, and the redistributions of REM sleep to the first half of the night (16). In dementia, sleep is fragmented and there is less deep sleep (17). Sleep apnea is more common in patients with Alzheimer's disease than in the general population and may be correlated with the severity of the dementia (18). Patients with schizophrenia have fragmented sleep, and those with panic disorder may have a panic attack during sleep, often during stages 2 or 3 (17).

Sleep Disorders Associated With a Medical Disorder

Numerous medical conditions interfere with sleep. These conditions include nocturnal cardiac ischemia, sleep-related asthma, pain syndromes, paroxysmal nocturnal dyspnea, gastroesophageal reflux disorder, and fibrositis. The latter two conditions are discussed here.

Gastroesophageal reflux disorder occurs exclusively in sleep. Patients may complain of sleep fragmentation, fatigue, and chest discomfort on awakening. Sleep-related gastroesophageal reflux is potentially more harmful than daytime reflux because of reduced swallowing and greater likelihood of aspiration. Some patients with nocturnal choking and sleep fragmentation may have reflux, and some apnea patients may have coexisting gastroesophageal reflux. Sleep problems usually resolve with treatment of the reflux.

Fibrositis (also known as fibromyalgia) is a chronic syndrome associated with a waxing-and-waning pattern with episodes of musculoskeletal pain, fatigue, and nonrestorative sleep. It occurs predominantly in women and usually appears in the third or fourth decade of life. Treatment is directed toward promotion of good sleep hygiene practices, exercise, and treatment with tricyclic antidepressants or selective serotonin reuptake inhibitor antidepressants. Treatment with the more sedating agents, such as amitriptyline and trazodone, is often successful in decreasing discomfort and promoting sleep.

■ TREATMENT

Table 9–3 lists clinical guidelines for sleep hygiene that are recommended for all of the disorders (19, 20). Some suggestions about the use of sedative-hypnotics are also mentioned here.

Use of Sedative-Hypnotics

Kupfer and Reynolds (21) have identified six basic tenets to follow when prescribing sleep medications (see Table 9–4).

Three benzodiazepines used as hypnotic agents are flurazepam, temazepam, and triazolam, although others, such as lorazepam and oxazepam, are often used for this purpose. These and other commonly used hypnotics are listed in Table 9–5 (22). Flurazepam is absorbed rapidly and has a long elimination half-life (19). If this drug is used repeatedly, the patient may experience daytime somnolence and memory impairment (21). The 15-mg dosage has been reported to be as effective as the 30-mg dosage (23). Temazepam has an intermediate elimination half-life and no active metabolites. Because it is absorbed slowly, it should be taken 30 minutes before bedtime (19). Triazolam has a short elimination half-life, and because of reports of anterograde amnesia, its use is not recommended here. Quazepam has a pharmacological profile similar to that of flurazepam (22).

Because benzodiazepine use can lead to dependence, other

TABLE 9–3. **Sleep hygiene recommendations**

Wake up at the same time every morning
Get regular exercise
Eat a light snack before bedtime
Avoid excessive noise, warmth, or cold
Avoid evening caffeine (remember that some medications contain caffeine)
Avoid alcohol before bedtime
Avoid tobacco use before bedtime
Do not read, eat, or watch TV in bed
Do not nap during the day
If you cannot fall asleep, turn on the light and do something else (e.g., read or watch TV) out of bed and preferably in another room

TABLE 9–4. **Guidelines for the use of hypnotics**

1. Use the lowest effective dosage
2. Use medications two or four times a week (instead of nightly)
3. Use medications on a short-term basis, for example, for 3–4 weeks[a]
4. Discontinue medications gradually
5. Anticipate that rebound insomnia may occur once the medication is stopped
6. Use medications with short elimination half-lives

Note. [a]Research trials of hypnotics have not been long enough to determine efficacy on a chronic basis (2).

TABLE 9–5. **Commonly used hypnotics**

Medication	Dosage (mg)
Flurazepam	15–30
Temazepam	15–30
Quazepam	7.5–15
Zolpidem	5–10
Trazodone	50–100
Melatonin	0.2–3

agents have been used as sedative-hypnotics. Zolpidem is less likely to cause cognitive side effects. However, because it acts at the gamma-aminobutyric acid (GABA) receptor complex, it may produce dependence and, thus, should be used for no more than 4 weeks (21). The tertiary amine tricyclic antidepressants, such as amitriptyline, have anticholinergic effects and can be lethal in overdosages. Trazodone, an antidepressant with serotonergic effects, is also commonly used, but no studies have demonstrated that antidepressants are effective in treating insomnia in the absence of a mood disorder (21).

Over-the-counter medications such as antihistamines help patients feel drowsy but do not induce sleep (24) and they impair daytime functioning (21). One study has demonstrated good results using melatonin in the elderly (25).

Generally, the decision to use sedative-hypnotics should be based on the patient's age and medical condition. All sleep medications, if taken regularly and at high dosages, and if active metabolites accumulate, will cause memory problems, falls, daytime somnolence, and accidents (21). The elderly (26), pregnant women, patients with sleep apnea, and patients with renal or hepatic disease are at greater risk for side effects (21). Table 9–6 lists hypnotics that have problematic side effects (22). These medications should be used as little as possible, if at all.

Other Treatments

Several psychological and behavioral techniques, such as biofeedback and progressive muscular relaxation, are available to help treat insomnia; they require referral to an experienced specialist to be effective.

■ CONCLUSION

Sleep disorders in the general population are common and may be easily overlooked. Many sleep disorders mimic medical and psychiatric conditions. Primary care practitioners, with appropriate

TABLE 9–6. **Hypnotics with troublesome side effects**

Medication class	Medication(s)	Side effects
Tricyclic antidepressants	Amitriptyline (Elavil) Imipramine (Tofranil) Doxepin (Sinequan)	Anticholinergic side effects; may cause confusion and delirium in the elderly
Antihistamines	Dyphenhydramine (Benadryl) Hydroxyzine (Vistaril)	Anticholinergic side effects; may cause confusion and delirium in the elderly
Barbiturates	Secobarbital (Seconal)	Lethal in overdosage; excessive central nervous system depression; potential for dependence
Nonbarbiturates	Chloral hydrate (Noctec) Glutethimide (Doriden)	Lethal in overdosage; confusion in the elderly
Benzodiazepines	Triazolam (Halcion)	Anterograde amnesia
Over-the-counter medications	Excedrin PM, Unisom	Do not induce sleep; impair daytime function

referral when indicated, will find that patients report an overall improvement in their health if their sleep symptoms are alleviated. Literature on sleep disorders may be obtained through the American Sleep Disorders Association, located in Rochester, Minnesota, at (507) 287-6006.

■ REFERENCES

1. Reynolds CF, Kupfer DJ: Sleep disorders, in The American Psychiatric Press Textbook of Psychiatry. Edited by Talbott JA, Hales RE, Yudofsky SC. Washington, DC, American Psychiatric Press, 1988, pp 737–752
2. Reynolds CF, Kupfer DJ: Neuropsychiatric aspects of sleep disorders, in The American Psychiatric Press Textbook of Neuropsychiatry. Edited by Hales RE, Yudofsky SC. Washington, DC, American Psychiatric Press, 1987, pp 241–256
3. Kales A, Vela-Bueno A, Kales JD: Sleep disorders: sleep apnea and narcolepsy. Ann Intern Med 106:434–443, 1987
4. Mitler MM: The multiple sleep latency test as an evaluation for excessive somnolence, in Sleeping and Waking Disorders. Edited by Guilleminault C. Menlo Park, CA, Addison-Wesley, 1982, pp 145–153
5. Guilleminault C, Van Den Hoed J, Mitler MM: Clinical overview of the sleep apnea syndromes, in Sleep Apnea Syndromes. Edited by Guilleminault C, Dement WC. New York, Alan R Liss, 1978, pp 1–12
6. Smallwood RG, Vitiello MV, Giblin EC, et al: Sleep apnea: relationship to age, sex, and Alzheimer's dementia. Sleep 6:16–22, 1983
7. Smith PL, Gold AR, Myers DA, et al: Weight loss in mildly to moderately obese patients with obstructive sleep apnea. Ann Intern Med 103:850–855, 1985
8. Issa FG, Sullivan CE: Alcohol, snoring, and sleep apnea. J Neurol Neurosurg Psychiatry 45:353–359, 1982
9. Dolly FR, Block AJ: Effect of flurazepam on sleep-disordered breathing and nocturnal oxygen desaturation in asymptomatic subjects. Am J Med 73:239–243, 1982
10. Lugaresi E, Cirignotta F, Montagna P: Snoring: pathogenic, clinical, and therapeutic aspects, in Principles and Practice of Sleep Medicine. Edited by Kryger MH, Roth T, Dement WC. Philadelphia, PA, WB Saunders, 1989, pp 494–500

11. Brownell IG, West P, Sweatman P, et al: Protriptyline in obstructive sleep apnea: a double-blind trial. N Engl J Med 307:1037–1042, 1982
12. Conway WA, Zonck F, Piccione P: Protriptyline in the treatment of obstructive sleep apnea. Thorax 37:49–53, 1982
13. Ancoli-Israel S, Kripke DF, Mason W, et al: Sleep apnea and nocturnal myoclonus in a senior population. Sleep 4:349–358, 1981
14. Ohanna N, Peled R, Rubin AH, et al: Periodic leg movements in sleep: effect of clonazepam treatment. Neurology 35:408–411, 1985
15. Mellick GA, Mellick LB: Management of restless legs syndrome with gabapentin (Neurontin) (letter). Sleep 19:224–226, 1996
16. Gold PW, Goodwin FK, Chrousos GP: Clinical and biochemical manifestations of depression: relation to the neurobiology of stress, part I. N Engl J Med 319:348–353, 1988
17. Nofzinger EA, Buysse DJ, Reynolds CF, et al: Sleep disorder related to another mental disorder (nonsubstance/primary): a DSM-IV literature review. J Clin Psychiatry 54:244–259, 1993
18. Reynolds CF, Kupfer DJ, Taska LS, et al: Sleep apnea in Alzheimer's dementia: correlation with mental deterioration. J Clin Psychiatry 46:257–261, 1985
19. Hauri PJ, Ester MS: Insomnia. Mayo Clin Proc 65:869–882, 1990
20. Bootzin RR, Nicassio P: Behavioral treatment of insomnia, in Progress in Behavior Modification, Vol 6. Edited by Hersen M, Eisler R, Miller P. New York, Academic Press, 1978, pp 1–45
21. Kupfer DJ, Reynolds CF: Management of insomnia. N Engl J Med 336:341–346, 1997
22. Schatzberg AF, Cole JO, DeBattista C: Manual of Clinical Psychopharmacology, 3rd Edition. Washington, DC, American Psychiatric Press, 1997
23. Boston Collaborative Drug Surveillance Program: a clinical evaluation of flurazepam. J Clin Pharmacol 12:217–220, 1972
24. Kales J, Tan T-L, Swearingen C, et al: Are over-the-counter sleep medications effective? All-night EEG studies. Curr Ther Res Clin Exp 13:143– 151, 1971
25. Garfinkel D, Laudon M, Nof D, et al: Improvement of sleep quality in elderly people by controlled-release melatonin. Lancet 346:541–544, 1995
26. Gillin JC, Byerley WF: The diagnosis and management of insomnia. N Engl J Med 322:239–248, 1990

10

EATING AND WEIGHT DISORDERS

Barbara J. Wingate, M.D.
John P. O'Reardon, M.D.
Thomas A. Wadden, Ph.D.

Eating has emotional and physiological consequences. Issues of self-control, self-esteem, taste, satiety, satisfaction, and sharing exist for everyone in relation to food. Eating disorders and weight disorders are often discussed together because of the obvious overlap between food intake and weight control. However, eating disorders and weight disorders differ in such important ways that discussing them together runs the risk of minimizing those differences. Psychological conflicts usually underlie the symptoms of the eating and weight disorders.

■ EATING DISORDERS

The two eating disorders we discuss here are anorexia nervosa and bulimia nervosa. In patients with these disorders, the control of food intake becomes a means by which they try to manage the anxiety in their daily lives. The anxiety may be unconscious. Factors involved in the development of these disorders include the following:

- Societal pressure to maintain a low weight
- Family history of obesity, eating disorders, affective disorders, and substance abuse

- Failure to master developmental tasks during puberty
- Family stressors (e.g., financial difficulties, divorce, and physical and/or sexual abuse)
- Membership in groups, including sports teams, in which chronic dieting is required

Patients with eating disorders are often reluctant to seek medical attention and often see clinicians only at the behest of their families.

Anorexia Nervosa

A cardinal feature of anorexia nervosa is the refusal to maintain body weight at or above a minimally acceptable level. The patient's weight is 15% or more below what would be expected based on height and age. Some dissatisfaction with body weight and shape is common in Western, especially American, culture, but it reaches an extreme level in the anorexic patient. The anorexic patient has a pronounced body image disturbance and, even when emaciated, perceives him- or herself as overweight. Even when malnourished, the patient has an intense fear of gaining weight and will interpret minor fluctuations in daily weight as an unacceptable loss of control. Female anorexic patients are amenorrheic (1). Table 10–1 lists the criteria for anorexia nervosa.

Anorexia nervosa has two subtypes: restricting and binge-eating/purging (1). Patients with the restricting type of anorexia nervosa are able to maintain daily food intake as low as 200–600 calories/day. Other anorexic patients are not able to rigidly control their intake by dieting and use binge-eating and purging behavior as a means of caloric regulation. Patients with this type of anorexia nervosa binge on food and then purge by vomiting, using diuretics or laxatives, or exercising excessively. The anorexic patient's weight is 15% or more below ideal weight.

Anorexia nervosa is a rare disorder. The female-to-male ratio is 10:1. It is seen more often in practices that include adolescent females, and it occurs frequently in urban settings. Comorbid psychi-

TABLE 10–1. **DSM-IV criteria for anorexia nervosa**

1. A deliberate weight loss or a deliberate failure to gain weight during an expected period of growth such that weight is less than 85% of ideal weight
2. Fear of gaining weight, even though underweight
3. Body image disturbance
4. Amenorrhea in female patients
5. Categorized as either the restricting or the binge-eating/purging type

Source. Adapted from American Psychiatric Association 1994 (1).

atric disorders are common, including major depression and obsessive-compulsive disorder.

Evaluation. The peak initial onset of anorexia nervosa occurs between ages 13 and 20 years, but its onset may occur as early as 6 years of age or as late as the fifth decade. Male patients are at risk of being underdiagnosed, and an eating disorder must be considered for those men who present with low weight or a body image misperception. Anorexic patients often exhibit a rapid weight loss of greater than 10% of total body weight in a 3-month period or, in younger children, a failure to thrive and to reach expected weight (1). Because the onset of weight loss is almost always connected to a distressing loss or perceived failure, a body image disturbance must be present for the practitioner to distinguish between anorexia and a loss of appetite associated with major depression.

When an eating disorder is suspected, the practitioner should ask questions relating to the topics listed in Table 10–2. These topics apply to the eating disorders and the weight disorders and can be discussed in the review of systems (2).

Because the anorexic patient is likely to exhibit denial, certain topics may be of higher yield in eliciting fear of fat and drive for thinness. For example, if the underweight patient is asked the weight at which he or she would be comfortable, the patient invari-

TABLE 10–2. **Topics to consider when evaluating patients with eating and weight disorders**

Weight fluctuation (highest/lowest/current)
Patient and family history of obesity, eating disorders, or other psychiatric illness
Daily food intake and types of food eaten
Menstrual history
Satisfaction with weight and body image
Purging behaviors and use of diet pills, laxatives, and diuretics
Amount, type, and purpose of exercise
Current psychosocial stressors

ably gives a weight well below the acceptable threshold. Body image disturbance is revealed by reports of feeling fat even when the patient obviously is not. The athlete may require additional evaluation to sort out special training needs, diet, and weight concerns.

Patients may complain of fatigue, constipation, abdominal pain or bloating, headaches, cold intolerance, depression, or sleep difficulties. In most patients, these problems will resolve with adequate nutrition and weight gain. Other medical causes of weight loss, emaciation, and gastrointestinal disturbances must be ruled out, and the differential diagnosis includes malignancies, endocrinological abnormalities, inflammatory bowel disease, malabsorption states, and peptic ulcer disease. The patient's age at onset will dictate the level of workup, because the differential diagnosis changes with age. The disturbed body image and continuing pursuit of thinness will be the key to eliminating excessive testing, particularly in high-risk female populations.

The physical examination most frequently shows emaciation. Many patients will exhibit orthostatic hypotension or bradycardia. Dermatological changes associated with starvation are frequently observed, including dry skin, brittle nails, and the emergence of lanugo-like hair. In the purging anorexic patient, the practitioner may also observe swelling of the parotid glands or, less frequently, callused knuckles, loss of enamel, and increased caries. Amenorrheic patients will develop osteopenia.

Table 10–3 lists some laboratory tests to use as part of the screening examination. These tests can also be used for patients with bulimia nervosa.

These studies frequently reveal anemia or thyroid abnormalities. Conditions that may require emergency intervention include hypokalemia, severe bradycardia, orthostatic hypotension, and electrocardiogram changes. Weight loss below 25% of ideal body weight is an indication for hospitalization, although it is harder to get authorization for this in many managed care plans (3).

Bulimia Nervosa

Bulimia nervosa, a disorder of binge eating and purging, is more common than is anorexia nervosa; its prevalence is 1%–2% (4). Patients with bulimia nervosa are most often female, and the age at onset is 18–21 years, although it can occur in the early teens. A binge is defined as a discrete period of uncontrollable and excessive eating (1). Between 500 and 5,000 calories can be consumed during a binge. Patients' weights vary widely. Bulimia nervosa has purging and nonpurging subtypes, but the majority of patients vomit. Studies estimate that 20%–45% of patients use laxatives once daily and that 15% use laxatives several times daily (5). In

TABLE 10–3. **Laboratory tests recommended for patients with eating disorders**

Electrolytes, blood urea nitrogen, and creatinine
Complete blood count
Calcium, magnesium, phosphate
Thyroid function tests
Liver function tests
Electrocardiography
Bone density test (if anorexia is diagnosed)

bulimia nervosa, there is a higher comorbidity of affective illness and substance abuse, particularly alcohol abuse, than there is in anorexia nervosa. Table 10–4 lists the diagnostic criteria for bulimia nervosa.

Evaluation. Bulimic patients are more likely than anorexic patients to seek help on their own. Because their purging behaviors are a source of shame, they may be secretive about their symptoms. The use of the screening topics listed in Table 10–2 is crucial. Because of the recurrent vomiting, patients may complain of esophageal or gastric irritation or bloody emesis.

The presence of bulimia nervosa will not be obvious on examination. Most patients will not be emaciated and will not necessarily be below normal weight. Although the practitioner may look for and find swollen parotid glands or callused knuckles, the diagnosis is rarely made this way. It may take more than one appointment for the patient to explain the symptoms. If the diagnosis remains uncertain, the practitioner should schedule a follow-up appointment within the next 1–2 months.

The laboratory workup is the same as for anorexic patients (see Table 10–3), although the bone density test may be unnecessary for bulimic patients. An elevated salivary gland amylase isoenzyme level is found in some patients. There is no corresponding rise in serum lipase levels as occurs in patients with pancreatitis. Despite significant binge eating and purging, the patient's electrolytes are often normal, helping to mask even severe illness. Laboratory re-

TABLE 10–4. **DSM-IV criteria for bulimia nervosa**

1. Recurrent episodes of binge eating
2. After a binge, various behaviors performed as an attempt to prevent weight gain—for example, induction of vomiting or use of laxatives
3. The binges and behaviors occur at least twice a week for 3 months
4. Categorized as either the purging or the nonpurging type

Source. Adapted from American Psychiatric Association 1994 (1).

sults cannot be used to make the diagnosis, but they are important in assessing the patient's progress during treatment.

■ TREATMENT OF EATING DISORDERS

General Principles

The primary care practitioner is often the first professional to acknowledge and diagnose an eating disorder. The manner in which the practitioner addresses the problem may set the tone and pace of the treatment process. There is a general consensus that normalized eating is the true cornerstone of recovery. The medical and underlying psychosocial issues must be addressed concomitantly, but the first issue to be addressed (barring an acute psychiatric crisis or medical emergency) must be nutritional rehabilitation. It is often not the first issue solved, but establishing it early as a priority is necessary. Most physicians are not well trained in the specifics of nutrition and do not have time to design an appropriate nutritional plan for their patients. Consultation with a nutritionist familiar with eating disorders is desirable. The American Anorexia Bulimia Association can help practitioners find specialists in eating disorders. The association is located in New York City and can be reached at (212) 575-6200.

Most specialists who treat eating disorders are committed to a team approach that recognizes the complexity of the illness and the need for multidisciplinary care. Those involved should be the primary care physician, a nutritional counselor, and a mental health professional. The primary care physician will often explain to the patient the need for multidisciplinary care and will be responsible for providing referrals to specialists. Addressing the physical complaints without ignoring psychosocial factors is the best role for the primary practitioner on the team.

When a comorbid psychiatric condition is present, the patient must be referred to a psychiatrist to determine the need for pharmacotherapy. Improperly treated psychiatric disorders will hinder the development of normal eating patterns. Psychotherapy is also often indicated. Cognitive-behavioral therapy is the most useful form of psychotherapy for the treatment of purging behaviors (6).

Anorexia Nervosa

The anorexic patient who is eating 300–600 calories/day will find it challenging to imagine the daily intake of 2,000–3,800 calories that is often required for weight gain. An initial plan, under the supervision of a nutritionist, should, within 1 week, have the patient consume a minimum of 1,000–1,500 calories/day. Incremental increases in caloric intake can be planned so that the patient gains 1–2.5 pounds per week (7). Rapid overfeeding should be avoided to minimize the risk of refeeding edema and to limit the patient's anxiety as he or she gains weight.

The patient will have a plethora of somatic complaints, some exaggerated by anxiety and body image distortion. The patient may complain of bloating, gas, uncomfortable fullness, constipation, diarrhea, and nausea. Imagine the discomfort the average person would feel if required to triple or quadruple daily food intake within 1 week. The task is challenging, but practitioners must encourage and demand progress. The restricting anorexic patient will need help expanding daily intake to include fats and proteins.

By definition, the (female) anorexic patient has become amenorrheic and is at risk for developing osteoporosis. A bone density scan is an essential tool for determining current loss of mineralization and continuing loss in patients with chronic or unremitting anorexia nervosa. Estrogen replacement may be indicated if the patient has a chronic condition or is not gaining weight in an agreed-upon time frame. The patient who is below 75% of ideal body weight, or who has had a rapid weight loss within 2–3 weeks, should be hospitalized for medical stabilization, nutritional rehabilitation, and psychological support. Under monitored situations, some patients may tolerate weight gains of up to 4 pounds per week. A specialized eating disorders program is optimal if available. If care is to be given in a general medical hospital or on a general psychiatric unit, the staff must be educated about nutritional goals and about providing firm but supportive monitoring.

Psychiatric medications are of little help in stimulating appetite. The depression that accompanies anorexia nervosa is frequently a result of starvation and improves with adequate weight and normalized eating. For patients with comorbid psychiatric illness, the full range of psychiatric medications and interventions must be used.

Bulimia Nervosa

Bulimic patients will likely have trouble with the notion of a normal meal plan of 1,800–2,200 calories/day and will greatly fear any plan that prevents purging. They will have a dread of weight gain. Initially they are likely to start food restriction behaviors and, if abusing laxatives, to escalate their misuse unless they receive supportive interventions. Bulimic patients may have significant nutritional deficiencies because of the poor quality of foods chosen (i.e., a preponderance of sweets and high-fat foods). The nutritionist's role is to design a meal plan that provides satisfying food, starting with a good breakfast. The therapist's role is to help patients devise more constructive ways of relieving anxiety and to help them understand the psychological conflicts that precipitate the binge eating and purging.

The purging subtype of bulimic nervosa has a low incidence of mortality, but if a patient is vomiting on a daily basis, misusing laxatives regularly, or experiencing comorbid depression with suicidality, he or she may require hospitalization for adequate stabilization and safety. Inpatient care is much harder to obtain through most managed care contracts. Day treatment and evening partial programs may be the best options available for the bulimic patient who is not suicidal. Many communities do not have specialized programs for the treatment of bulimia nervosa.

Psychiatric medications have a significant role in the treatment of bulimia nervosa. The importance of antidepressants in conjunction with cognitive therapy is well documented (5). The selective serotonin reuptake inhibitors (SSRIs) and tricyclic antidepressants are effective. Bupropion should be avoided because bulimic patients are at risk for seizures when taking this medication (8).

■ WEIGHT DISORDERS

Obesity is not a psychiatric disorder, but a subset of obese patients have what is currently called binge-eating disorder. In this disorder, patients will uncontrollably consume large quantities of food. Unlike bulimic patients, they do not purge or exercise, and as a result of the overeating, they become obese (1). These patients tend to be female, but the prevalence is divided between the genders more evenly than in anorexia nervosa or bulimia nervosa. Patients with binge-eating disorder also have a poorer success rate at weight loss, are more likely to end treatment prematurely, and have a higher incidence of major depression than do those obese patients who are not binge eaters (9).

Much has been written on the etiology of the increased prevalence of obesity in the United States. High-fat diets and decreased physical activity account for the vast majority of cases, but other factors include genetics (10), individual history of weight gain (e.g., after a pregnancy), medications (e.g., anticonvulsants, antipsychotics, lithium, and antidepressants), and other medical conditions (e.g., rheumatoid arthritis leading to inactivity and weight gain). Obesity places an individual at risk for medical conditions such as diabetes, coronary artery disease, hypertension, sleep apnea, osteoarthritis, and gall bladder disease.

Obesity and *overweight* are different terms, although they frequently overlap and are often used interchangeably. However, all overweight persons are not obese. Weight recommendations are generally based on standards set by the 1983 Metropolitan Life Insurance tables, which remain controversial. Obesity is defined not only by weight standards but also by the ratio of body fat to weight. The best way to determine obesity is by the calculation of body mass index (BMI), which is the ratio of weight in kilograms to height in meters squared. Generally, overweight is defined as a BMI of 25 to 30, and obesity is defined as a BMI over 30.

■ TREATMENT OF WEIGHT DISORDERS

Between 90% and 95% of patients who lose weight will regain it (9). Losing weight is beneficial for patients who are mildly or moderately obese and who also have other medical conditions such as diabetes or hypertension, but it is not clear whether losing weight is helpful for obese patients without these conditions (11). Therefore, the goal of treatment is to decrease morbidity, not to achieve thinness (12).

Medications alone are not effective, although some medications deserve mention. A common side effect of the SSRIs is appetite suppression. When these medications are used to treat depression, weight loss can result that can persist for up to 6 months (9). The combination of fenfluramine (Pondimin), an SSRI, or its metabolite, dexfenfluramine (Redux), with phentermine, a sympathomimetic, gained attention as a treatment for obesity. However, fenfluramine has been associated with pulmonary hypertension, and various combinations of these three agents have been associated with valvular heart disease (12). As a result, fenfluramine and dexfenfluramine have been removed from the market. Surgery is recommended for severe obesity, defined as a BMI greater than 40 (13). For obese binge-eating patients, cognitive therapy is helpful in eliminating binges (9).

■ CONCLUSION

The eating disorders are anorexia nervosa, bulimia nervosa, and binge-eating disorder. The weight disorder of obesity is not a psychiatric disorder. The focus of treatment for eating disorders is to achieve normalized food intake, and that for obesity is to decrease associated morbidity. Because there may be psychiatric comorbidity with the eating disorders, psychiatric referral is often necessary for recovery.

REFERENCES

1. American Psychiatric Association: Diagnostic and Statistical Manual of Mental Disorders, 4th Edition. Washington, DC, American Psychiatric Association, 1994
2. Powers PS: Initial assessment and early treatment options for anorexia nervosa and bulimia nervosa. Psychiatr Clin North Am 19:701–703, 1996
3. Kaye WH, Kaplan AS, Zucker MC: Treating eating disorders in a managed care environment. Psychiatr Clin North Am 19:793–810, 1996
4. Fairburn CG, Agras WS, Wilson GT: The research on the treatment of bulimia nervosa: practical and theoretical implications, in The Biology of Feast and Famine: Relevance to Eating Disorders. Edited by Anderson GH, Kennedy SH. New York, Academic Press, 1992
5. Gwirtsman HE: Laxative and emetic use in bulimia nervosa, in Special Problems in Managing Eating Disorders. Edited by Yager J, Gwirtsman HE, Edelstein JC. Washington, DC, American Psychiatric Press, 1992, pp 145–162
6. Mitchell JE, Raymond N, Specker S: A review of the controlled trial of pharmacotherapy and psychotherapy in the treatment of bulimia nervosa. Int J Eat Disord 14:229–247, 1993
7. Rock CL, Curran-Celentano J: Nutritional management of eating disorders. Psychiatr Clin North Am 19:701–713, 1996
8. Horne RL, Ferguson JM, Pope HG, et al: Treatment of bulimia with bupropion: a multi-center controlled trial. J Clin Psychiatry 49:262–266, 1988
9. Wadden TA: The treatment of obesity: an overview, in Obesity: Theory and Therapy. Edited by Stunkard AJ, Wadden TA. New York, Raven, 1993
10. Stunkard AJ, Sorensen TIA, Hanis C, et al: An adoption study of human obesity. N Engl J Med 14:193–198, 1986
11. Kassirer JP, Angell M: Losing weight—an ill-fated New Year's resolution. N Engl J Med 338:52–54, 1998
12. Rosenbaum M, Leibel RL, Hirsch J: Obesity. N Engl J Med 337:396–407, 1997
13. Brownell KD, Fairburn CG (eds): Eating Disorders and Obesity: A Comprehensive Handbook. New York, Guilford, 1995

11

SUICIDE AND VIOLENCE

E. Cabrina Campbell, M.D.
Stephan C. Mann, M.D.
Michael F. Gliatto, M.D.
Sheryl D. Hunter, M.D.

■ SUICIDE

Suicide is the ninth leading cause of death in the United States (1). Although a relatively rare event, a patient's suicide is devastating to both the family and the practitioner. Suicidality exists as a spectrum ranging from fleeting thoughts of death to completed suicide. An understanding of the epidemiology and demographics of suicide is crucial when clinically assessing the patient who has suicidal ideation. Table 11–1 lists selected risk factors for suicide (1–3).

Men are three times more likely than women to commit suicide (1). In general, the suicide rate increases with age; the highest overall rate is among persons age 65 or older. In men, the rate rises steadily and peaks after age 75, whereas in women, the rate peaks by the late 40s to early 50s (1). Recent increases in the suicide rate have been noted in young men and women between the ages of 15 and 24 (1).

Whites commit suicide more often than do African Americans, although the rate for African Americans is increasing. Suicide is not a leading cause of death among Hispanic or Asian Americans. Rates for American Indians and Alaskan Natives are higher than the national rate (1).

The presence of a social support system appears to provide pro-

TABLE 11–1. **Risk factors for suicide**

Demographics	
	Gender (male)
	Age (> 65 years)
	Race (Caucasian, Native American, Alaskan Native)
	Marital status (divorced or widowed)
	Geographical area (western states)
	Religion (protestant)
Psychiatric history	
	Family history
	History of suicide attempt
	Social stressor(s)
	Psychiatric disorder
Other	
	Seasonal factors
	Medical illness

tection against suicide. Individuals who are widowed or divorced have a higher suicide rate than do those who are single, and those who are married have the lowest suicide rate (2).

Across all age groups, the use of firearms ranks first as the method by which both men and women kill themselves. Hanging and drug overdosage rank second for men and women, respectively (1). Suicide occurs most frequently in the western mountain states and least often in the mid-Atlantic region (1). Religious affiliation is important: Protestants have the highest suicide rate, followed by Jews and then Catholics (2).

More suicides occur during spring and early summer than during other times of year. A family history of suicide is associated with an increased risk of completed suicide as is an individual history of attempted suicide. Other risk factors for suicide include the presence of physical illness and the occurrence of stressful life events such as unemployment, bereavement, and a change of residence (1). Psychiatric disorders associated with suicide are discussed in the next section.

Patients who attempt suicide have a demographic profile different from those who complete suicide: the former are younger (aged 25–44 years [4]), are female, and use overdosing or cutting instead of firearms (1). Substance abuse is frequently involved in suicide attempts (3).

Psychiatric Disorders

More than 95% of patients who commit suicide have a psychiatric disorder at the time of death (3). Table 11–2 lists the most consistently reported disorders (1, 2). These disorders are often comorbid (5). For instance, panic disorder per se has not been identified as increasing a patient's risk for suicide, but it does when the disorder is comorbid with major depression or alcohol abuse (5). Patients with schizophrenia are not prone to commit suicide during periods of psychosis (though this can certainly happen), but they are prone to do so during periods of remission, when they are more likely to feel hopeless and depressed (4). According to one study, alcoholic patients who have undergone a recent loss of a relationship, and hence are susceptible to depression, are at an increased risk for suicide (6).

Medical Disorders

A number of medical illnesses (e.g., cancer, multiple sclerosis, and spinal cord injury) are associated with a greater risk of suicidality (7). However, most of the patients with these disorders who did

TABLE 11–2. **Psychiatric disorders associated with an increased risk for suicide**
Major depression
Substance abuse
Schizophrenia
Borderline personality disorder
Panic disorder

commit suicide also had a psychiatric disorder, most notably major depression or alcohol abuse (7). One study found that the risk for suicide is not increased among human immunodeficiencly virus (HIV)–positive patients in a variable period (from 15 days to 98.5 months) following HIV screening but that the risk increases after symptomatic disease develops (8).

Evaluation

Most patients who complete suicide have never been evaluated by a mental health professional. However, many patients who commit suicide have seen a primary care practitioner in the month prior to their deaths (9). Of those patients who do commit suicide, two-thirds have made prior attempts, although this history is rarely obtained by the nonpsychiatric practitioner (9). Patients with psychiatric disorders, particularly the disorders mentioned earlier in this chapter; patients with chronic debilitating illnesses; and patients with recent stressors should be asked periodically about suicidal ideation.

The mnemonic SAD PERSONS may help practitioners remember the risk factors and clinical symptoms to include in a thorough assessment of suicidal patients (10). Tables 11–3 and 11–4 outline the mnemonic and its use in facilitating treatment planning. These are guidelines only and cannot be used as a substitute for a complete evaluation.

Another useful method of assessing for suicide risk is to make a checklist of short-term risk factors (defined as risk factors for completed suicide occurring within 1 year of the initial assessment) and long-term risk factors (defined as risk factors for completed suicide occurring more than 1 year after the initial assessment) (11, 12). Long-term risk factors include feelings of hopelessness, family history of suicide, history of poor impulse control, unemployment, and the epidemiological factors listed in Tables 11–1 and 11–3 (12). Table 11–5 lists the short-term risk factors (11, 12); if present, these factors require immediate attention, as discussed in the next section.

TABLE 11–3. **The SAD PERSONS scale**

Sex	Assign 1 point if patient is male, 0 points if female
Age	Assign 1 point if patient is 19 or younger or 45 or older
Depression	Assign 1 point if present
Previous attempt	Assign 1 point if present
Ethanol abuse	Assign 1 point if present
Rational thinking loss	Assign 1 point if patient is psychotic
Social supports lacking	Assign 1 point if lacking, especially if loss is recent
Organized plan	Assign 1 point if plan is made and method lethal
No spouse	Assign 1 point if patient is divorced, widowed, separated, or single
Sickness	Assign 1 point if present, especially if sickness is chronic, debilitating, or severe

Source. Adapted from Patterson et al. 1983 (10).

Treatment

In this section, we provide some general guidelines for treatment of suicidal ideation. These guidelines parallel those indicated in Table 11–4.

1. If the patient has only occasional thoughts of suicide and is able to state that he or she can refrain from hurting him- or herself and can contact the practitioner should he or she feel worse, then the practitioner should schedule a series of frequent follow-up appointments. Psychiatric disorders should be treated accordingly.
2. If the patient has thought of a plan but is hesitant to put it into effect, then the practitioner should ascertain the patient's level of intent to die (e.g., a will has been written or rewritten, a sui-

TABLE 11–4. **Scoring and treatment planning using the SAD PERSONS scale**

Total points	Treatment plan
0–2	Send home with follow-up
3–4	Send home with close follow-up; consider hospitalization
5–6	Strongly consider hospitalization; depending on confidence in the follow-up arrangement
7–10	Hospitalize or commit

Source. Adapted from Patterson et al. 1983 (10).

TABLE 11–5. **Short-term risk factors for suicide**

Panic attacks
Anxiety
Anhedonia
Alcohol abuse
Impaired concentration
Insomnia
Recent (within 3 months) discharge from psychiatric hospital

Source. Adapted from Simon 1998 (12).

cide note has been written, or lethal means are available). Family members should be enlisted to help the practitioner dissuade the patient from suicide and to engage in the treatment plan. A psychiatric consultation should be obtained, and psychiatric treatment should be initiated. Hospitalization should be considered.

3. If the patient has a plan, is determined to die, and has access to lethal means, then the patient should be hospitalized. The patient should not be left alone. The patient may not permit the practitioner to contact family members; however, when a patient's life or that of another is threatened, confidentiality may be breached.

The patient may also refuse to go to an emergency room or crisis center to be evaluated for admission. Each state has its own laws regarding involuntary commitment to psychiatric facilities. The staff at a crisis center will be familiar with these laws and can guide the practitioner on the proper steps to take to get the patient to the crisis center. The police sometimes have to be called. The commitment process itself should be performed by mental health professionals.

4. A suicidal patient who is intoxicated, has a history of serious suicide attempts, is psychotic, or is not well known by the practitioner should be safely transported to a psychiatrist, local crisis center, or emergency room.

Medications

The suicidal patient who has symptoms of major depression should not take tricyclic antidepressants, because they can be lethal in overdosages. Likewise, such a patient should not take low-potency neuroleptics. The agents discussed in Chapter 1 are safe to use. Because a time lag exists between initiation of medication therapy and onset of clinical improvement, the patient will require frequent follow-up appointments to monitor suicidality. The risk for suicide may increase as the patient's energy level improves (13).

Because patients who are anxious or sleepless are at an increased risk for suicide (11), these symptoms should be addressed immediately. The practitioner can dispense a limited supply (e.g., enough to last until the next appointment) of a sedating benzodiazepine (see Chapters 2 and 9), which would not be fatal in an overdosage unless ingested with other central nervous system depressants such as alcohol.

■ VIOLENCE

Homicide rates have generally been stable for the past 25 years, but the rates of homicide and violent behavior committed by adolescents and young adults have been increasing (14). Violence is more prevalent among men (14), but in psychiatric patients, the association of gender and violence is not clear (15). Poverty and nonwhite race place an individual at increased risk for being a victim of violence (14). The most lethal injuries are a result of the use of guns (14).

Violence in Patients With Psychiatric Disorders

It has been suggested that those with mental illnesses are prone to violent behavior. One of the most thorough studies addressing this issue was a component of the Epidemiologic Catchment Area surveys (16). Individuals with Axis I disorders had a prevalence of violent behavior four times that of community residents with no mental disorders. Individuals with alcohol and drug abuse had rates of violence 10–15 times that of the general population. Those with anxiety disorders, mood disorders, and schizophrenia had rates of violence five to six times higher than those among the general population. Individuals with more than one diagnosis (e.g., the combination of schizophrenia and alcohol abuse) had rates of violent behavior greater than would be expected by simply adding the individual rates. Among the Axis II disorders, antisocial personality disorder had a rate of violence as high as that of substance abuse (15).

Another risk factor for committing violence is a history of violence (17). Individuals with a history of violence have the following personality characteristics: hostility, paranoid ideation, and interpersonal sensitivity. Hostility includes being aggressive, resentful, and irritable. Paranoid ideation is not the same as a paranoid delusion; it refers to a general sense that others are unfriendly and that they cannot be trusted. Interpersonal sensitivity refers to an exaggerated feeling of social inferiority, that is, that one's personal attributes are not as good as those of another (18).

Psychotic symptoms are also associated with violence. These symptoms include well-systematized paranoid delusions, such that one is able to organize and implement a plan to harm the perceived persecutor (17, 19); delusions that one is controlled by outside forces; delusions of thought insertion; and delusions of being followed (20).

Another characteristic noted in patients with homicidal behaviors is a history of suicide attempts (18). Many patients who had homicidal ideation (without carrying out the act) also had suicidal ideation (18). This observation suggests a link between aggression directed at others and that directed toward the self (18). The family history of violent patients includes aggression, suicide attempts, and completed suicides (18).

Although alcohol is implicated in a majority of violent crimes (21), other substances, such as the hallucinogens and phencyclidine (PCP) (22) and cocaine and amphetamines (23), also have been associated with violence. Table 11–6 summarizes the risk factors for violent behavior.

Table 11–7 lists other neuropsychiatric disorders associated with aggression (24).

Evaluation

A patient is unlikely to arrive in the outpatient clinic threatening violence. However, if such a situation occurs, the practitioner should not attempt to do an evaluation. Maintaining the safety of patient, practitioner, and staff is the priority, and the police should be called immediately.

TABLE 11–6. **Risk factors for violent behavior**
History of violence
Substance abuse
Antisocial personality disorder
Mood disorder, anxiety disorder, schizophrenia
Psychotic symptoms
Hostility and other personality traits
History of suicide attempts
Family history of violence

TABLE 11–7. **Neuropsychiatric disorders associated with aggression**
Brain injury
Dementia
Huntington's disease
Mental retardation
Seizure disorder
Personality disorders

If, during an evaluation for another symptom, a patient reveals that he or she is homicidal or has problems with aggression, the practitioner must determine whether immediate referral to a crisis center or an emergency room is indicated or whether the psychiatric consultation can be deferred for a few days. As when evaluating suicidal patients, the practitioner should be conservative and take appropriate measures to ensure the safety of both the patient and potential victims. If a patient tells the practitioner about a specific plan to hurt someone, the practitioner has a legal responsibility to warn and to protect the potential victim. This responsibility is part of the *Tarasoff* decision of 1976.

However, to fulfill the requirements of the *Tarasoff* decision, the practitioner needs to conduct a thorough evaluation of the patient's risk for homicidal behavior. This assessment is beyond the purview of a generalist and should not be pursued without consulting a psychiatrist. If the patient admits to homicidal ideation or if the patient seems dangerous (e.g., intoxicated, psychotic, agitated, and/ or belligerent), the crisis center or emergency department should be contacted and the steps outlined earlier in this chapter for treatment of suicidal ideation should be followed. Some patients with homicidal ideation will require involuntary admission to a psychiatric facility.

In an outpatient setting, practitioners are more likely to see victims of abuse than assaultive patients. All states mandate reporting cases of abuse of children and the developmentally disabled (17). Suspicion of child abuse is sufficient to notify the proper authorities (25). The abuse of the elderly is probably underreported; 46 states currently mandate reporting cases of elder abuse (26).

Domestic Violence

Domestic violence is defined as violence between adults who are in an intimate relationship (17). Most of the victims are women, and a majority of the women are not living with or married to the men who abuse them (27).

When battered women seek treatment, it often is not for the injuries sustained. Rather, they may have nonspecific complaints such as headaches, sleep disturbances, or anxiety. Table 11–8 lists the situations that require a screen for physical abuse (27).

Most states require practitioners to report serious injuries (e.g., gunshot wounds) (28). The practitioner should advise the patient to seek legal counsel, which is available through various community organizations. Staff members at these organizations can help the patient decide whether a restraining order or assault and battery charges are necessary (27). If the patient or her children are in imminent danger, she should be referred to the city or county human services agency immediately.

Treatment

Table 11–9 lists several medications that have been used to treat aggression (29). These medications should be used only in consultation with a psychiatrist.

TABLE 11–8. **Situations requiring a screen for physical abuse**
Repeated vague somatic complaints
Pregnancy
Miscarriage or abortion
Poorly explained injuries
Suicidality or history of suicide attempts
Visit to practitioner is said to be someone else's idea

TABLE 11–9. **Medications used to treat aggression**

Medication	Clinical use
Carbamazepine	Use if electroencephalogram is abnormal, especially if temporal lobe focus is present
Lithium	Use in patients in whom aggression is secondary to mania
Antipsychotics	Use only for short-term management of aggression; long-term use associated with tardive dyskinesia
Benzodiazepines	Use only for short-term management
β-blockers	Use when aggression is secondary to brain injury, mental retardation, or other central nervous system processes
Trazodone	Use in aggression secondary to Alzheimer's disease

■ CONCLUSION

Because suicide and violence are difficult to predict, a thorough evaluation of suicidality and violence often requires a consultation with mental health professionals. Legal issues are involved concerning the safety of the patient and others; these issues also should be addressed by psychiatrists or lawyers. The primary care practitioner should be familiar with the risk factors associated with suicide and violence so that he or she can determine when an emergency referral should be made.

■ REFERENCES

1. Moscicki EK: Identification of suicide risk factors using epidemiologic studies. Psychiatr Clin North Am 20:499–517, 1997
2. Cavanaugh S: The diagnosis and treatment of depression in the medically ill, in Manual of Psychiatric Consultation and Emergency Care. Edited by Guggenheim F, Weiner M. New York, Jason Aronson, 1994, pp 211–222

3. Hirschfeld RMA, Russell JM: Assessment and treatment of suicidal patients. N Engl J Med 337:910–915, 1997
4. Fawcett J, Clark DC, Busch KA: Assessing and treating the patient at risk for suicide. Psychiatric Annals 23:244–255, 1993
5. Henriksson MM, Aro HM, Marttunen MJ, et al: Mental disorders and comorbidity in suicide. Am J Psychiatry 150:935–940, 1993
6. Murphy GE, Armstrong JW Jr, Hermele SL, et al: Suicide and alcoholism: interpersonal loss confirmed as a predictor. Arch Gen Psychiatry 36:65–69, 1979
7. Mackenzie TB, Popkin MK: Suicide in the medical patient. Int J Psychiatry Med 17:3–22, 1987
8. Dannenberg AL, McNeil JG, Brundage JF, et al: Suicide and HIV infection: mortality follow-up of 4,147 HIV-seropositive military service applicants. JAMA 276:1743–1746, 1996
9. Murphy GE: The physician's responsibility for suicide, II: errors of omission. Ann Intern Med 82:305–309, 1975
10. Patterson WM, Dohn HH, Bird J, et al: Evaluation for suicidal patients: the SAD PERSONS scale. Psychosomatics 24:343–349, 1983
11. Fawcett J, Scheftner WA, Fogg L, et al: Time-related predictors of suicide in major affective disorder. Am J Psychiatry 147:1189–1194, 1990
12. Simon RI: Concise Guide to Psychiatry and Law for Clinicians, 2nd Edition. Washington, DC, American Psychiatric Press, 1998
13. Malone K: Pharmacotherapy of affectively ill suicidal patients. Psychiatr Clin North Am 20:613–624, 1997
14. Stanton B, Baldwin RM, Rachuba L: A quarter century of violence in the United States: an epidemiologic assessment. Psychiatr Clin North Am 20:269–282, 1997
15. Asnis GM, Kaplan ML, Hundorfean G, et al: Violence and homicidal behaviors in psychiatric disorders. Psychiatr Clin North Am 20:405–425, 1997
16. Swanson JW, Holzer CE, Ganju VK, et al: Violence and psychiatric disorder in the community: evidence from the Epidemiologic Catchment Area surveys. Hospital and Community Psychiatry 41:761–770, 1990
17. Resnick PJ, Scott CL: Legal issues in treating perpetrators and victims of violence. Psychiatr Clin North Am 20:473–487
18. Asnis GM, Kaplan ML, van Praag HM, et al: Homicidal behaviors among psychiatric outpatients. Hospital and Community Psychiatry 45:127–132, 1994

19. Wessely S, Buchanan A, Reed A: Acting on delusion, I: prevalence. Br J Psychiatry 163:69–76, 1993
20. Link BG, Stueve CA: Psychotic symptoms and the violent/illegal behavior of mental patients compared to community controls, in Violence and Mental Disorders: Developments in Risk Assessment. Edited by Monahan J, Steadman H. Chicago, IL, University of Chicago Press, 1994, pp 137–159
21. Murdoch D, Pihl RO, Ross D: Alcohol and crimes of violence: present issues. International Journal of the Addictions 25:1065–1081, 1990
22. Budd RD, Lindstrom DM: Characteristics of victims of PCP-related deaths in Los Angeles County. J Toxicol Clin Toxicol 19:997–1004, 1982
23. Honer WE, Gewirtz E, Turey M: Psychosis and violence in cocaine smokers. Lancet 2:451, 1987
24. Fava M: Psychopharmacologic treatment of pathologic aggression. Psychiatr Clin North Am 20:427–451, 1997
25. Kaplan SJ: Physical abuse of children and adolescents, in Family Violence: A Clinical and Legal Guide. Edited by Kaplan SJ. Washington, DC, American Psychiatric Press, 1996, pp 1–35
26. Brewer RA, Jones JS: Reporting elder abuse: limitations of statutes. Ann Emerg Med 18:1217–1221, 1989
27. Sassetti MR: Domestic violence. Prim Care 20:289–305, 1993
28. Bryant WG, Panico S: Physicians' legal responsibilities to victims of domestic violence. N C Med J 55:418–421, 1994
29. Yudofsky SC, Silver JM, Schneider SE: Pharmacologic treatment of aggression. Psychiatric Annals 17:397–407, 1987

INDEX

Page numbers printed in **boldface** *type refer to tables or figures.*

Acetaminophen, 59, **60**
Acetylcholine, 78, 80, 86–87
Acquired immunodeficiency syndrome (AIDS), 75. *See also* Human immunodeficiency virus
Acute stress disorder, **27**
Adjustment disorders, 32–33
Adrenal glands, 111
Adrenocorticotropic hormone, **114**
Advanced sleep phase syndrome, 178–179
African-Americans
  depression and, 9
  suicide and, 199
Age and age at onset. *See also* Children; Elderly
  dementia and, 77
  eating disorders and, 188,189, 191
  generalized anxiety disorder and, 32
  melancholic depression and, 3
  obsessive-compulsive disorder and, 31
  schizophrenia and, 116
  sleep patterns and, 169, 170
  social phobia and, 30
  suicide and, 199
Aggression, and violent behavior, 207, **208, 210**
Agitation, medications for, **88,** 89
Agoraphobia
  social phobia and, 30
  panic disorder with, 26, **27,** 29
Agranulocytosis, 130
Akathisia, and antipsychotics, 126–127
Alcohol and alcohol abuse. *See also* Substance abuse
  benzodiazepine abuse and, 69
  dementia secondary to, 81
  depressive symptoms and, 4
  drug interactions and, **60**
  intoxication and, **54–55**
  sleep disorders and, 177–178
  substance-induced psychotic disorder and, **114**
  suicide and, 201
  treatment of, 53, 58–60, 64–65
  violent behavior and, 207
  withdrawal and, **56–57, 114**
Alcoholics Anonymous, 61, 157
Alprazolam
  anxiety disorders and, 34, **40,** 44
  substance use disorders and, **63,** 69

Alzheimer's disease
dementia and, 77, 78, 80, 81, 85, 86, 89
sleep disorders and, 180
Amantadine, 127
Amenorrhea, 194
American Academy of Family Physicians, **66**
American Academy of Neurology, 83
American Anorexia Bulimia Association, 193
American Cancer Society, **66**
Amitriptyline
depression and, 17
sexual function and, 162
sleep disorders and, 181, 183, **184**
Amphetamines
sleep disorders and, 177
substance-induced psychotic disorder and, **114**
violent behavior and, 207
Anabolic steroids, and substance-induced psychotic disorder, **114**
Analgesics, and substance-induced psychotic disorder, **113**
Anorexia nervosa
body dysmorphic disorder and, 97–98
characteristics of, 188
DSM-IV criteria for, **189**
evaluation of, 189–191
treatment of, 194–195
Anorgasmia, 161
Antiandrogens, 157
Antibiotics, and substance-induced psychotic disorder, **113**
Anticholinergics, and psychotic disorders, **113, 114,** 125, 127, 129
Anticipatory anxiety, 26
Anticonvulsants
sleep disorders and, 177
substance-induced psychotic disorder and, **113**
Antidepressant medications. *See also* Tricyclic antidepressants
atypical depression and, 3
bipolar disorder and, 5
dysthymia and, 6
elderly and, 21
major depression and, 10–11
melancholic depression and, 3
nicotine withdrawal and, 68
psychotic depression and, 3
sexual function and, 153
Antihistamines, 183, **184**
Antihypertensive agents
major depression and, **6**
side effects of, 152–153
substance-induced psychotic disorder and, **113**
Anti-inflammatory agents, and major depression, **6**
Antimalarial agents, and substance-induced psychotic disorder, **113**
Antineoplastics, and substance-induced psychotic disorder, **113**
Antioxidant agents, 86
Antiparkinsonian dopamine agonists, **113**
Antipsychotic medications
aggression and, **210**
cognitive disorders and, 89

psychotic depression and, 3, 14
psychotic disorders and, **113,** 121–126
side effects of, **123–124,** 126–130
Antisocial personality disorder, 99, 206
Antituberculous medications, and substance-induced psychotic disorder, **113**
Anxiety. *See also* Anxiety disorders
benzodiazepines and, 18
depression and symptoms of, 9
eating disorders and, 187, 194
monoamine oxidase inhibitors and, 17
Anxiety disorder due to general medical condition, 33–34
Anxiety disorders. *See also* Anxiety
characteristic symptoms of, **27–28**
comorbidity and, 35–36
definition of, 25
diagnosis of, 25–26
restless legs syndrome and, 176
substance abuse and, 36
treatment of
generalized anxiety disorder, 43–44
general principles of, 36–37
medications for, **38–40**
obsessive-compulsive disorder, 42–43
panic disorder, 37, 41
social phobia, 41–42
specific phobia, 41
stress disorders, 44
types of
adjustment disorders and stress disorders, 32–33
anxiety disorder due to general medical condition, 33–34
generalized anxiety disorder, 31–32
obsessive-compulsive disorder, 31
panic disorder, 26, 29
phobias, 29–30
substance-induced anxiety disorder, 34–35
violent behavior and, 206
Apnea. *See* Obstructive sleep apnea
Apolipoprotein E (APOE), 80
Appointments. *See also* Follow-up visits
initial visits and doctor-patient relationship, 141–144
psychotic disorders and, 120–121
treatment of depression and, 18
Arousal disorder in women, 157–158
Astemizole, 14, 16
Atypical depression, 3, 11
Auditory hallucinations, 108
Autoimmune disorders
conditions associated with major depression, **5**
neuroleptic malignant syndrome and, 128
psychosis due to, **111**
Autonomic system, and substance abuse, **54, 56**
Avoidant personality disorder, 30

Babinski reflex, 176
Baclofen, **113**
Barbiturates
  alcohol and, **60**
  side effects of as sleep medications, **184**
  substance abuse and, **54–57,** 73–74
Basal ganglia diseases, 110
Behavior
  cognitive disorders and, 87–90
  factitious disorder and bizarre, 99
  psychotic disorders and disorganized, 109
  styles of and doctor-patient relationship, 135–138, **139,** 144–145
  violent behavior, 205–210
Behavioral therapy. *See also* Cognitive-behavioral therapy
  sexual disorders and, 156, 157
  stress disorders and, 44
Benzisoxazoles, **124**
Benzodiazepines
  aggression and, **210**
  alcohol and, 59, **60**
  anxiety disorders and, 36, 37, **40,** 43–44
  cognitive disorders and, 89
  depression and, 17–18
  mania and, 6
  psychotic disorders and, 127
  sexual function and, 153
  sleep disorders and, 176, 178, 180, 181, **182,** 183, **184**
  substance use disorders and, **54–57,** 68–71, 74
  suicidal ideation and, 205
Bereavement, 6–7
Beta-blockers
  aggression and, **210**
  anxiety disorders and, 42
  psychotic disorders and, 127
  sexual function and, 153
Binge eating, 188, 196
Biopsychosocial perspective, on treatment of anxiety disorders, 36
Bipolar disorder, 4–6, 10, 15
Bizarre delusions, 108
Blocking, and thought disorders, 108
Blood alcohol content (BAC), 58, **59**
Body dysmorphic disorder, **94,** 97–98
Body image, and anorexia nervosa, 188, 189, 190, 194
Body mass index (BMI), 196–197
Borderline personality disorder, **201**
Brain
  Alzheimer's disease and neuroanatomy of, 78, 80
  dementia and lesions of, **79**
  injury of and violent behavior, **208**
Breast-feeding, and antipsychotics, 130
Brief psychotic disorder, 118
Bromide, **114**
Bromocriptine, 128, 177
Bulimia nervosa
  characteristics of, 191–192
  DSM-IV criteria for, **192**
  evaluation of, 192–193
  treatment of, 195–196

Bupropion
depression and, **12,** 15–16
sexual function and, 153
substance use disorders and, **62,** 67, 68
Buspirone
anxiety disorders and, **38,** 43, 44
cognitive disorders and, 89
Butalbital, 73
Butyrophenones, **123**

Caffeine, 34, 177
Cancer chemotherapy, 75
Cannabis. *See* Marijuana
Carbamazepine
aggression and, **210**
bipolar disorder and, 5
cognitive disorders and, 89
Carbidopa, 176
Carbohydrate deficient transferrin (CDT), 58, **59**
Carbon dioxide, as toxin, 112, **114**
Carbon monoxide, 112, **114**
Cardiovascular medications, and major depression, **6**
Cataplexy, 173
Catatonia, 109, 117
Central nervous system
anticholinergic medications and, 129
infection of as cause of dementia, **79**
major depression and disorders of, **5**
medications precipitating major depression, **6**
Cerebral cortex, and subcortical dementias, 80
Cerebrospinal fluid, neural thread protein levels and Alzheimer's disease, 80
Children. *See also* Age and age at onset
abuse of and reporting requirements, 208–209
sleep patterns and, 169, 179
Chloral hydrate, **184**
Chlordiazepoxide, **40**
Chlorpromazine
dementia and, **88**
psychotic disorders and, 122, **123,** 130
Chlorprothixene, **123**
Chronic obstructive pulmonary disease (COPD), 59
Cigarettes, 65
Cimetidine, **113**
Circadian rhythm disorder, **172** 178–179
Circumstantiality, and thought disorders, 108
Clomipramine
anxiety disorders and, 37, **38,** 42, 43
body dysmorphic disorder and, 98
sexual disorders and, 162
Clonazepam
anxiety disorders and, **40,** 42, 43–44
sleep disorders and, 176, 178, 180
substance use disorders and, **63**
Clonidine, **63,** 153
Clozapine, **124,** 125, 130

Cocaine
  intoxication and, **54–57**
  substance-induced psychotic disorder and, **115**
  treatment of substance abuse and, 72–73
  violent behavior and, 207
Cognitive-behavioral therapy. *See also* Behavioral therapy; Psychotherapy
  for anxiety disorders, 41, 42
  for eating disorders, 194
  for sexual disorders, 156, 157, 163
  for weight disorders,197
Cognitive disorders. *See also* Dementia
  evaluation of, 82–86
  general principles, 77
  rare forms of, 81–82
  treatment of, 86–90
  types of
    Alzheimer's disease, 78, 80
    dementia secondary to alcoholism, 81
    subcortical dementias, 80–81
    vascular dementia, 80
Cognitive distortions, and specific phobia, 41
Combat experience, and posttraumatic stress disorder, 33
Combination trials, of medications for depression, 20
Combined therapy, for anxiety disorders, 41
Comorbidity, with other psychiatric disorders
  anxiety disorders and, 35–36
  eating disorders and, 188–189, 192, 193–194
  somatic disorders and, 102
Compliance, of patient with treatment
  depression and, 18
  psychotic disorders and, 120, 126
  substance use disorder and, 64
Compulsions, definition of, 31
Consultation. *See* Psychiatrists
Continuous positive airway pressure (CPAP), 174
Conversion disorder, **94,** 96
Creutzfeldt-Jakob disease, 81, 82
Culture. *See also* Society
  eating disorders and, 188
  sexual disorders and, 151
Cyclic guanosine monophosphate (GMP), 159
Cytochrome P450 drug-metabolizing enzymes, 14

Dantrolene, 128
Death, from complications of Alzheimer's disease, 78, 80. *See also* Suicide and suicidal ideation
Delayed sleep phase syndrome, 178, 179
Delirium
  anxiety and, 36
  dementia and, 85–86
Delirium tremens (DTs), 58, 61
Delta sleep, 169
Delta-9-tetrahydrocannabinol (THC), 74–75

Delusional disorders. *See also* Delusions
of psychotic type, 118
of somatic type, **94,** 100
Delusions. *See also* Delusional disorder
delusional disorder and, 100
general characteristics of, 107–108
medications for, **88**
psychotic depression and, 2–3
selective serotonin reuptake inhibitors and, 11, 14
violence and, 206–207
Demanding behavioral style, and doctor-patient relationship, 136, 137, **139**
Dementia. *See also* Cognitive disorders
causes of, **79**
characteristics of, 77
comorbidity with depression in elderly, 21
misdiagnosis of melancholic depression as, 3
potentially reversible or irreversible types of, 78
secondary to alcoholism, 81
sleep and, 180
violent behavior and, **208**
Dementia of depression, 85
Demographics, and risk factors for suicide, **200,** 201
Denial, and anorexia nervosa, 189
Dental appliances, and sleep disorders, 175
Dependent behavioral style, and doctor-patient relationship, 136, **139**
Depression. *See also* Major depression
anorexia nervosa and, 195
course and prognosis of, 7–8
dementia and comorbidity with, 89
DSM-IV criteria for, 1, **2**
evaluation of, 8–9
geriatric patients and, 21
incidence of, 1
suicidal patients and, 22
treatment of
guidelines for, 18–19
medication and, 10–18, 19–20
nonpharmacological, 20
primary care practitioners and, 9–10
resistance to, 19–20
types of
atypical depression, 3
bereavement, 6–7
bipolar disorder, 4–6
dysthymia, 6
melancholic depression, 3
postpartum depression, 4
psychotic depression, 2–3
seasonal depression, 3
secondary depression, 4
Desipramine, 17
Detoxification
alcohol abuse and, 59–61
benzodiazepines and, 70–71
Dexfenfluramine, 197
Diagnosis. *See also* Differential diagnosis; Evaluation
of anxiety disorders, 25–26
of obsessive-compulsive disorder, 31

Diagnosis *(continued)*
- of panic disorder, 26
- of substance abuse, **51**
- of substance dependence, 49, **50**
- uncertain and doctor-patient relationship, 138, 140, 141, 144

Diazepam
- anxiety disorders and, 34, **40,** 43
- side effects of, 70

Dibenzothiazepines, **124**
Dibenzoxazepines, **123, 124**
Diet, and monoamine oxidase inhibitors, 17, 41. *See also* Nutrition
Differential diagnosis. *See* Diagnosis; Evaluation
Difficult patients, and doctor-patient relationship, 137–138
Diffuse Lewy body disease, 81
Dihydroindolones, **123**
Diphenylbutylpiperidines, **124**
Disordered thought processes, 108–109
Disorganized type, of schizophrenia, 117
Dissociative disorders, 116
Disulfiram, **62,** 64, **114**
Diuretics, and sexual function, 153
Diurnal variation, and melancholic depression, 3
Doctor-patient relationship. *See also* Health care system; Primary care practitioners; Therapeutic alliance
- patient variables and, 135–141
- somatoform and related disorders and, 100–104
- suggestions on development and maintenance of, **139,** 141–146
- treatment of depression and, 20

Domestic violence, 209
Donepezil, 87
Dopaminergic agonists, 176–177
Dosages, of medications for
- anxiety disorders, 37, **38, 41,** 43
- cognitive disorders, 87
- depression, 11, **12–13,** 16, 20
- psychotic disorders, **123–124,** 125, 131
- sleep disorders, 181, **182**
- substance use disorders, 61, **62–63**

Doxepin, **184**
Dreams, 179
Dronabinol, 75
Drug holidays, and selective serotonin reuptake inhibitors, 14
Drug-induced sexual dysfunction, 153
Drug interactions
- alcohol and, 58–59, **60**
- monoamine oxidase inhibitors and, 17, 41
- tricyclic antidepressants and, 42

DSM-IV
- definition of traumatic stressor, 32–33
- diagnostic criteria for
  - anorexia nervosa, **189**
  - anxiety disorders, 25
  - bulimia nervosa, **192**
  - depression, 1, **2**
  - manic episode, **7**
  - phobia, 29

schizophrenia, 116, **117**
somatization disorder, 96
substance abuse, **51**
substance dependence, 49, **50**
Dyphenhydramine, **184**
Dyspareunia, 162–163, 164
Dysthymia, 6

Eating disorders
anorexia nervosa
characteristics of, 188
evaluation of, 189–191
treatment of, 194–195
bulimia nervosa
characteristics of, 191–192
evaluation of, 192–193
treatment of, 195–196
general principles, 187–188, 193–194
Education
doctor-patient relationship and, 138, 146
treatment of depression and, 18
Elderly. *See also* Age and age at onset
abuse of, 209
anticholinergics and, 129
antipsychotics and, 125
benzodiazepines and, 68
dementia and, 77, 83
depression and, 9, 14, 15, 17, 21
diazepam and, 43
panic disorder and, 29
sexual disorders and, 160, 164
sleep disorders and, 175, 178, 183
substance-induced anxiety disorder and, 34–35
Electroconvulsive therapy (ECT), for depression, 3, 20
Endocrine disorders
as cause of dementia, **79**
major depression and, **5, 6**
psychosis due to, 111
sexual disorders and, 158
Epilepsy, and pseudoseizures, 96
Essential vulvodynia, 163
Estrogen replacement therapy
Alzheimer's disease and, 86
anorexia nervosa and, 194
sexual disorders and, 156, 158, 163
Evaluation. *See also* Diagnosis
of anorexia nervosa, 189–191
of bulimia nervosa, 192–193
of cognitive disorders, 82–86
of depression, 8–9
of psychotic disorders, 119
of sexual disorders, 150–153
of sleep disorders, 170
of suicidal ideation and suicide risk, 202, **203**
of violent behavior, 207–209
Exposure and response prevention, and obsessive-compulsive disorder, 43
Extrapyramidal side effects (EPS), and antipsychotics, 122, 125, 126–127, 131
Eyes
antipsychotics and, 129
intoxication and, **54**
withdrawal and, **56**

Factitious disorder, **94,** 98–99
Family. *See also* Family history
Alzheimer's disease and, 90
treatment of suicidal ideation and, 204

Family history
of depression and Alzheimer's disease, 85
risk factors for suicide and, 200
violent behavior and, 207
Female orgasmic disorder, 160–161
Fenfluramine, 197
Fibrositis, 181
Firearms, 200, 206
Flashbacks, 33
Flight of ideas, and thought disorders, 108–109
Flumazenil, 71
Fluoxetine
anxiety disorders and, 37, **38,** 41, 43
body dysmorphic disorder and, 98
dementia and, **88,** 89
depression and, 11, **12,** 15
dosage of, 20
Fluphenazine, and psychotic disorders, 122, **123, 124,** 126
Flurazepam, 181, **182**
Fluvoxamine
anxiety disorders and, **38,** 43, 44
dosage of, **12**
termination of, 19
Follow-up visits
doctor-patient relationship and, 144–146
somatic and related disorders and, 102
treatment of depression and, 18
Frontal lobe dementias, 81–82
Gabapentin, 177
Gastroesophageal reflux disorder, 180
Gastrointestinal system, and substance abuse, **55, 56**
Gender
depression and, 9
eating disorders and, 188, 189, 191
sexual function and, 150
suicide and, 199
violence and, 206
Generalized anxiety disorder
agitated depression and, 35
characteristics of, **27,** 31–32
treatment of, 43–44
Genetics, of Alzheimer's disease, 78, 80
Geriatric patients. *See* Elderly
GIDDINESS (mnemonic), 5
Glaucoma, 75, 129
Glucocorticoids, and substance-induced psychotic disorder, **114**
Glutamyl transferase (GCT) levels, 58, **59**
Glutethimide, **184**
Grandiose delusions, 107
Guidelines, for treatment
of depression, 18–19
of sleep disorders with hypnotics, **182**
of substance use disorders, 52–53
of suicidal ideation, 203–205

Hallucinations
general characteristics of, 108
medications for, **88**
psychotic depression and, 2–3

Hallucinogens, **115,** 207
Haloperidol
dementia and, **88**
psychotic disorders and, 122, **123, 124,** 125, 126, 129
Head trauma, 119
Health care system. *See also* Doctor-patient relationship; Primary care practitioners
factitious disorder and, 98–99
societal cost of depression, 1
somatoform disorders and, 94–95
Heat stroke, and antipsychotics, 129
Heavy metals, 112, **114**
High-dose dependence, and benzodiazepines, 69
Homicide, 205
Homosexuality, and sexual disorders, 161, 164–165
Hormones. *See* Endocrine disorders; Estrogen replacement therapy; Testosterone
Hospitalization
for bipolar disorder, 10
for depression, 10
for eating disorders, 191, 194–195
for postpartum depression, 4
for psychotic disorders, 120
for substance use disorders, 52, 71
for suicidal ideation, 204–205
for violent behavior, 208
Hostility, and violence, 206
Human immunodeficiency virus (HIV). *See also* Acquired immunodeficiency syndrome
dementia and, 83, 165
homosexuality and safe sex practices, 202
psychotic disorders and, 119
risk for suicide and, 202
Huntington's disease, 80, 110, **208**
Hydroxyzine, **184**
Hyperarousal, 33
Hyperprolactinemia, and antipsychotics, 129
Hyperthermia, and neuroleptic malignant syndrome, 128
Hyperthyroidism, 111
Hypoactive sexual desire disorder, 156
Hypoalbuminemia, 86
Hypochondriasis, **94,** 97
Hypomania, and bipolar disorder, 4, 5
Hypnotics, and sleep disorders, **182**
Hypopnea, 174
Hypothyroidism, 110, 111

Illusions, and hallucinations, 108
Imipramine
anxiety disorders and, 37, **38,** 44
depression and, 17
sleep disorders and, **184**
Impotence, 158–160
Infanticide, and postpartum psychosis, 4
Infections
dementia and, **79,** 82
psychosis and, 110

Inhalants, and substance abuse, **115**
Insecticides, 112, **114**
Insight-oriented therapy, and sexual disorders, 157
Insomnia, and selective serotonin reuptake inhibitors, 14. *See also* Sleep disorders
Interpersonal sensitivity, and violence, 206
Intoxication, signs and symptoms of, **54–55**
Intracavernous injections, for impotence, 159
Involuntary commitment, and suicidal ideation, 205
Irreversible dementia, 78

Jet lag, 178

Kegel exercises, 158

Laboratory tests
- for anorexia nervosa, 191
- for bulimia nervosa, **192**
- for cognitive disorders, 83, **85**
- for neuroleptic malignant syndrome, 128
- for psychotic disorders, 119
- for sexual disorders, 153, **155**
- for substance use disorders, 58, **59**

Language, and evaluation of sexual disorders, 151
Laser-assisted uvulopalatoplasty (LAUP), 175
Leaden paralysis, and atypical depression, 3
L-Dopa, 176
Lewy bodies, 81
Life stressors, and doctor-patient relationship, 138
Light therapy, 3, 179
Lithium carbonate
- aggression and, **210**
- anxiety disorders and, 43
- bipolar disorder and, 5
- cognitive disorders and, 89
- combination trials with antidepressants, 20

Liver function
- side effects of antipsychotics and, 130
- substance use disorders and tests of, 58, **59,** 64

Liver injury, and alcoholism, 59
Living situation, and substance use disorders, 52
Loosening of associations, and thought disorders, 108
Lorazepam
- anxiety disorders and, **40,** 43
- sleep disorders and, 178
- substance use disorders and, 60–61

Low-dose dependence, and benzodiazepines, 68–69
Loxapine, 122, **123**

Major depression. *See also* Depression
- bereavement and, 7
- cognitive disorders and medications for comorbid, **88**
- comorbidity with panic disorder, 35
- dementia and symptoms of, 83, 85
- diagnosis of, 7, 9

incidence of, 1
as lifelong disorder, 7–8
medications precipitating, **6**
postpartum depressions meeting severity levels for, 4
smoking and, 68
suicide and, **201**
Male erectile disorder, 158–160
Male orgasmic disorder, 161–162
Malingering, **94,** 100, 103–104
Mania
bipolar disorder and episodes of, 4–5
DSM-IV criteria for episodes of, **7**
psychotic symptoms and, 6
Marijuana
intoxication and, **54–55**
substance-induced psychotic disorder and, **114**
withdrawal from, **56–57**
Marital status, and suicide, 200
Marital therapy, and sexual disorders, 156
Mean corpuscular volume (MCV), 58, **59**
Medical conditions
anxiety disorder due to, 33–34
conversion disorder and, 96
depression and, 4, **5,** 14, 19
panic-like symptoms due to, 29
sexual disorders and, 156, 158, 164
sleep disorders associated with, 180–181
substance use disorders and, 52, 53, 58
suicide and, 201–202
Medications. *See also* Dosages; Drug holidays; Drug interactions; Side effects; Treatment; Specific types
as cause of delirium, 86
as cause of dementia, **79**
marijuana as, 74–75
precipitation of major depression by, **6**
psychosis associated with, 109–112, **113–115**
sexual function and, 152–153
treatment of
aggression, **210**
anxiety disorders, **38–40**
bulimia nervosa, 195–196
dementia, **88**
depression, 10–18, 19–20
psychotic disorders, 121–126, 130–131
sexual disorders, 158
somatic and related disorders, 102–103
substance use disorders, **62–63,** 64–65
suicidal ideation, 205
weight disorders, 197
Medroxyprogesterone acetate, 157
Melancholic depression, 3
Melatonin, **182,** 183
Memory, and dementia, 77, 80
Menopause, and sexual disorders, 158, 163
Mental retardation, and violent behavior, **208**
Mesoridazine, 122, **123,** 129
Metabolic disorders
as cause of dementia, **79**
psychosis due to, **111**

Methadone, 73
Methylphenidate, 21, 173
Mini-Mental State Exam (MMSE), 82–83, **84**
Mirtazepine
  depression and, 16
  dosage of, **13**
Mixed anxiety-depressive disorder, 35
Mixed episodes, of mania and depression in bipolar disorder, 5
Molindone, and psychotic disorders, 122, **123,** 128
Monoamine oxidase inhibitors (MAOIs)
  anxiety disorders and, 36, 37, 41–42
  consultation of psychiatrists on use of, 10
  depression and, 3, 17
Mood, and symptoms of substance abuse, **55, 56**. *See also* Mood disorders
Mood-congruent psychotic symptoms, 3
Mood disorders, 1. *See also* Depression; Mood
  bipolar disorder and, 4–6
  evaluation of by primary care practitioners, 8
  psychosis and, 112, 116
  secondary to medical condition or substance abuse, 4, **5**
  socioeconomic variables and reporting of symptoms, 9
  violent behavior and, 206
Mood-stabilizing medications, and bipolar disorder, 5, 6
Multidisciplinary care, for eating disorders, 193
Munchausen syndrome, 99

Naltrexone, and substance use disorders, **62,** 64–65
Narcolepsy, 171, **172,** 173
National Alzheimer's Association, 90
National Cancer Institute, **66**
National Institute of Aging, 83
National Institute of Mental Health, 83
National Institute of Neurological and Communicative Disorders and Stroke, 83
Native Americans, and suicide, 199
Nefazodone
  dementia and, **88**
  depression and, 16
  dosage of, **12,** 16
Neologisms, and thought disorders, 109
Nerve gas, 112, **114**
Neural thread protein, and Alzheimer's disease, 80
Neuroimaging
  dementia and, 83
  psychotic disorders and, 119
Neuroleptic malignant syndrome, 128
Neuroleptic medications
  anxiety disorders and, 43
  bipolar disorder and, 6
  cognitive disorders and, 88
  delusional disorder and, 100
  neuroleptic malignant syndrome, 128
  suicidal ideation and, 205

Neurological disorders, and psychosis, 110–111. *See also* Neuropsychiatric disorders
Neuromotor symptoms, of substance abuse, **54, 56**
Neuropsychiatric disorders, and violent behavior, **208.** *See also* Neurological disorders
Neuropsychological testing, for cognitive disorders, 83
Neurotransmitters
  Alzheimer's disease and, 78, 80
  sexual function and, 150
Nicotine, **62,** 65–68
Nightmares, 179
Night terrors and sleep terrors, 29, 179
Nocturnal panic attacks, 26, 29
Non-rapid eye movement (NREM) sleep, 169 170
Nortriptyline, 17
Numbing response, 33
Nursing staff, and doctor-patient relationship, 146
Nutrition. *See also* Diet
  as cause of dementia, **79**
  psychosis due to disorders of, **111**
  substance abuse and, **55, 56,** 60
  treatment of eating disorders and, 193, 194, 195

Obesity, 196–197
Obsessions, definition of, 31
Obsessive-compulsive disorder, **27,** 31, 35
Obstructive sleep apnea, **172,** 173–175
Occupational functioning, and intoxication, **55**
Olanzapine
  dementia and, **88,** 89
  psychotic disorders and, **124,** 131
Opiates, and substance abuse
  alcohol and, **60**
  intoxication and, **54–55**
  treatment of, 72
  withdrawal and, **56–57**
Organophosphate insecticides, 112, **114**
Orgasm and orgasmic disorders, 150, 160–162
Osteoporosis, 194
Outcome, of treatment for substance use disorders, 61, 64, 68
Overdosages
  of barbiturates, 74
  of benzodiazepines, 71
Overweight, definition of, 196, 197
Oxazepam
  anxiety disorders and, **40,** 43, 44
  substance use disorders and, 60–61, **62**

Pain. *See also* Pain disorders
  opiate abuse and, 72
  pain disorder and, 98
Pain disorders, **94,** 98, 162–163. *See also* Pain
Panic attacks, 26, 29
Panic disorder
  characteristics of, 26, **27**
  prevalence of, 29
  sleep disorders and, 180
  suicide and, **201**
Paranoid ideation, and violence, 206

Paranoid type, of schizophrenia, 117
Parasomnias, 179–180
Parathyroid glands, disorders of, 111
Parkinsonism, antipsychotic drug-induced, 127
Parkinson's disease, 80, 81, 110
Paroxetine
  anxiety disorders and, 37, **38,** 43
  dementia and, **88,** 89
  depression and, 11, **12,** 15, 19, 21, 20, 35
Patient. *See* Compliance; Doctor-patient relationship; Patient history
Patient history
  risk factors for suicide and, **200**
  sexual disorders and, 150–152
  substance use disorders and, 50–51
  violence and, 206–207
Pavor nocturnus, 179
Penile prostheses, and impotence, 160
Pentobarbital, **63**
Pergolide, 177
Periodic limb movements, **172,** 175–177
Perphenazine, 122, **123**
Persecutory delusions, 107
Personality disorders
  psychosis and, 116, 118
  violent behavior and, **208**
Pesticides, 112, **114**
Phencyclidine (PCP), 74, **115,** 207
Phenelzine, **38,** 41, 42
Phenobarbital, **63**
Phenothiazines, **60, 123**
Phentermine, 197
Phenytoin, **60**
Phobias, 29–30
Phototherapy, 179
Physical abuse, screening for, **209**
Physical examination
  anorexia nervosa and, 190–191
  cognitive disorders and, 82
Pick's disease, 81
Pimozide
  psychotic disorders and, 122, **124,** 129
  sexual disorders and, 153, **154**
  somatic delusions and, 100
Podophyllin, **114**
Polysomnography, and sleep disorders, 173, 174, 176
Position therapy, and sleep disorders, 174–175
Postpartum depression, 4
Postpartum psychosis, 4, 118
Posttraumatic stress disorder (PTSD)
  characteristics of, **27,** 33
  psychotic symptoms and, 116
  recurrence of symptoms of, 44
  substance abuse and, 35
Potentially reversible dementia, 78
Poverty of thought, 108
Pregnancy, and antipsychotics, 130
Premature ejaculation, 162
Prescription medications, abuse of, 34, 72
Prevalence
  of anxiety disorders, 25
  of bipolar disorder, 5
  of bulimia nervosa, 191
  of dementia, 77
  of generalized anxiety disorder, 32

of major depression, 1, 35
of obsessive-compulsive disorder, 31
of panic disorder, 29
of postpartum depression, 4
of schizophrenia, 116
of social phobia, 30
Primary care practitioners. *See also* Doctor-patient relationship; Health care system
diagnosis and treatment of sexual disorders by, 150–152
evaluation of mood disorders by, 8
prescriptions for benzodiazepines and, 68
psychotic disorders and, 119–121
smoking cessation and, 65, 66
treatment of depression by, 1, 9–10, 20, 21
treatment of eating disorders by, 193–194
Primary snoring, **172**
Prions, 82
Propranolol
anxiety disorders and, **38,** 42
cognitive disorders and, 89
psychotic disorders and, 127
substance use disorders and, 71
Prostaglandin E1, 159
Protriptyline, 175
Pseudodementia, 21, 85
Pseudoseizures, 96
Psychiatric disorders. *See also* specific disorders
as cause of dementia, **79**
psychosis associated with, 112, 116
sleep disorders associated with, 180
suicide and, 201
uncertain diagnoses and doctor-patient relationship, 138, 140, 144
violence in patients with, 206–207
Psychiatrists
consultations with on psychoactive medications
anxiety disorder and, 37
cognitive disorders and, 89–90
eating disorders and, 193–194
psychotic disorders and, 119–120, 125
coordination of care between generalists and, 145
referrals to
for cognitive disorders, 88
for depression, 10
for somatic and related disorders, 103
for suicidal ideation, 22
Psychomotor symptoms, of substance abuse, **54, 56**
Psychophysiological insomnia, 170–171, **172**
Psychosis. *See also* Psychotic disorders
associated with medical condition, 109–112
cognitive disorders and symptoms of, 87–90
definition of, 107
postpartum, 4, 118
violence and, 206–207

Psychosocial factors. *See also* Society; Support systems
 doctor-patient relationship and problems related to, 138, 140–141, 142
 somatic disorders and stressors, 103
Psychostimulants, and narcolepsy, 173
Psychotherapy. *See also* Cognitive-behavioral therapy; Treatment
 for depression, 20
 for eating disorders, 194
 for sexual disorders, 156
Psychotic depression, 2–3, 11, 14, 20
Psychotic disorders. *See also* Psychosis
 evaluation of, 119
 general characteristics of, 107–109
 primary care practitioners and, 119–121
 psychosis associated with medical condition, 109–112
 psychosis associated with psychiatric disorder, 112, 116
 schizophrenia, 36, 116–117, 120, 125–126, 180, **201,** 206
 treatment of, 121–126, 130–131
Purging, and eating disorders, 188, 195

Quazepam, 181, **182**
Quetiapine, **124,** 131

Race, and suicide, 199
Rapid eye movement (REM) sleep, 169–170, 180
Reactive mood, and atypical depression, 3
Recurrence. *See also* Relapse
 of depression, 8, 19
 of postpartum psychosis, 4
Reference, delusions of, 107–108
Referrals. *See* Psychiatrists
Rehabilitation, and substance use disorders, 52, 61, 64
Relapse. *See also* Recurrence
 depression and, 8, 18–19
 psychotic disorders and, 120, 125–126
 smoking cessation and, 67
 social phobia and, 42
Religious beliefs
 sexual disorders and, 161
 suicide and, 200
REM behavior disorder, 180
Restless legs syndrome, **172,** 175–177
Retinitis pigmentosa, 129
Risk factors
 for depression, 8, **9**
 for suicide, **200, 204**
Risperidone
 dementia and, **88,** 89
 psychotic disorders and, **124,** 130–131

SAD PERSONS (mnemonic), 202, **204**
Schizoaffective disorder, 118
Schizoid personality disorder, 30

Schizophrenia
anxiety and psychotic episodes, 36
general principles, 116–117
maintenance of antipsychotic drug treatment, 125–126
primary care practitioners and, 120
sleep disorders and, 180
suicide and, **201**
violent behavior and, 206
Schizophreniform disorder, 118
Screening
for physical abuse, **209**
for psychiatric disorders in primary care office, 144
for sexual dysfunction, **152**
Seasonal depression, 3
Seasonality, of suicide, 200
Secobarbital, **184**
Secondary depression, 4, **5,** 8
Sedative-hypnotics
sleep disorders and, 171, 181, **182,** 183
substance-induced psychotic disorder and, **115**
Seizures and seizure disorders
antipsychotics and, 128
benzodiazepines and, 70
bupropion and, 15–16
clozapine and, 130
psychosis and, 110
violent behavior and, **208**
Selective serotonin reuptake inhibitors (SSRIs)
anxiety disorders and, 36, 37, 41, 42, 43
bulimia nervosa and, 196
cognitive disorders and, 89
depression and, 3, 10, 11, 14–15, 20, 21
elderly and, 21
sexual disorders and, 157
weight disorders and, 197
Selegiline, 86
Self-destructive behavior, and doctor-patient relationship, 136, **139**
Self-help groups, and sexual disorders, 157
Sensory symptoms, of substance abuse, **54, 55**
Serotonergic agents, and premature ejaculation, 162
Sertraline
anxiety disorders and, **38,** 41, 43
dementia and, **88,** 89
depression and, 11, **12,** 14, 15, 20, 21
Sex addiction, 156, 157
Sexual arousal disorders, 157–160
Sexual aversion disorder, 156–157
Sexual desire disorders, 155–157
Sexual disorders. *See also* Sexual dysfunction
evaluation of, 150–153
general principles, 149
healthy sexual function, 149–150
special populations and, 164–165
types of and recommendations for treatment
male erectile disorder, 158–160
orgasmic disorders, 160–162
pain disorders, 162–163

Sexual disorders *(continued)*
types of and recommendations for treatment *(continued)*
sexual arousal disorders, 157–160
sexual desire disorders, 155–157
Sexual dysfunction. *See also* Sexual disorders
antipsychotics and, 129
screening for, **152**
Sexual phobia, 157
Side effects, of medications
antihypertensives, 152–153
antipsychotics, 122, **123–124,** 125, 126–130
bupropion, 15–16
disulfiram, 64
donepezil, 87
monoamine oxidase inhibitors, 41
neuroleptics, 88
olanzapine, 131
quetiapine, 131
risperidone, 131
selective serotonin reuptake inhibitors, 14, 15, 37, 41
sleep medications, 183, **184**
tetrahydroaminoacridine, 87
tricyclic antidepressants, 17
venlafaxine, 16
SIG: E CAPS (Mnemonic), 1, **2**
Sildenafil, 159–160
Skin
side effects of antipsychotics and, 129
symptoms of intoxication and, **55**
Sleep. *See also* Sleep disorders
efficiency of, 170
hygiene, 171, **182**
inventory, 170, **171**
latency, 177
medications for dementia and disturbance of, **88,** 89
nightmares and sleep terrors, 179
panic attacks and, 26, 29
substance abuse and, **57**
Sleep disorders. *See also* Insomnia; Sleep
evaluation of, 170**172,**
general principles, 169–170
treatment of, **172,** 181–183
types of
associated with medical disorder, 180–181
associated with psychiatric disorder, 180
circadian rhythm disorder, **172,** 178–179
narcolepsy, 171, 173
obstructive sleep apnea, **172,** 173–175
parasomnias, 179–180
periodic limb movements, **172,** 175–177
primary snoring, **172**
psychophysiological insomnia, 170–171, **172**
restless legs syndrome, **172,** 175–177
substance-related sleep disorders, **172,** 177–178
upper airway resistance syndrome, **172,** 174–175
Sleepwalking, 179

Social functioning. *See also* Society
- doctor-patient relationship and, 138
- intoxication and, **55**

Social phobia, **27,** 29–30, 41–42

Society. *See also* Culture; Psychosocial factors; Social functioning
- cost of depression to, 1
- sexual disorders and, 161, 164–165
- socioeconomic variables and reporting of mood symptoms, 9

Somatic delusions, 107

Somatic symptoms, of panic disorder, 26

Somatization disorder, **94,** 95–96

Somatizing behavioral style, and doctor-patient relationship, 136, 137, **139,** 142

Somatoform disorders
- general principles, 93–95
- types of
  - body dysmorphic disorder, **94,** 97–98
  - conversion disorder, **94,** 96
  - hypochondriasis, **94,** 97
  - pain disorder, **94,** 98
  - somatization disorder, **94,** 95–96

Somatosensory amplification, 97

Specific phobia, 29, 41

Stimulant-dependent sleep disorder, 177

Stress, and doctor-patient relationship, 138

Stress disorders, 32–33

Subcortical dementias, 80–81

Substance abuse. *See also* Alcohol and alcohol abuse; Substance use disorders
- anxiety disorders and, 34–35, 36
- benzodiazepines and, 18
- definition of, 49–50
- diagnosis of, **51**
- intoxication and, **54–55**
- motives for, 49
- psychotic disorders and, 109, 112, **113–115**
- resistance to treatment and, 19
- secondary depression, 4
- sleep disorders and, 177–178
- suicide and, 201
- violent behavior and, 206, 207
- withdrawal and, **56–57**

Substance dependence, 49, **50**

Substance-induced anxiety disorders, 34–35

Substance-induced psychotic disorders, 109, 112, **113–115**

Substance-related sleep disorders, **172** 177–178

Substance use disorders. *See also* Substance abuse
- general principles, 49–51
- treatment of
  - alcoholism, 53, 58–60, 64–65
  - barbiturates and, 73–74
  - benzodiazepines and, 68–71
  - cocaine and, 72–73
  - guidelines for, 52–53
  - hallucinogens and, 74–75
  - heroin and, 73
  - marijuana and, 74–75
  - medications for, **62–63**

Substance use disorders *(continued)*
treatment of *(continued)*
nicotine addiction, 65–68
opiates and, 72
Suffering behavioral style, and doctor-patient relationship, 136, 137, **139**
Suicide and suicidal ideation. *See also* Death
depression and, 8, 22
evaluation of, 202, **203**
general principles, 199–200
medical disorders and, 201–202
medications and, 205
postpartum psychosis and, 4
psychiatric disorders and, 201
risk factors for, **200, 204**
substance abuse and, 61, 71, 201
treatment of, 203–205
violent behavior and history of attempts, 207
Sundowning, and behavioral symptoms of cognitive disorders, 87
Support system. *See also* Psychosocial factors
substance use disorder and, 52
suicide risk and, 199–200
Surgery
severe obesity and, 197
sleep disorders and, 175

Tangentiality, and thought disorders, 108
Tarasoff decision (1976), 208
Tardive dyskinesia, and antipsychotics, 126, 127–128
TEACH (mnemonic), **50**
Temazepam
dementia and, **88**
sleep disorders and, 176, 178, 181, **182**
Terfenadine, 16
Testosterone, 150, 156, 164
Tetrahydroaminoacridine, 86–87
Therapeutic alliance, and somatoform disorders, 101. *See also* Doctor-patient relationship
Thiamine, 60
Thiazide, 153
Thienobenzodiazepines, **124**
Thioridazine, and psychotic disorders, 122, **123,** 129
Thiothixene, **123**
Thought, psychotic disorders and disordered processes of, 108–109
Thyroxine, and substance-induced psychotic disorder, **114**
Time zone change syndrome, 178
Tobacco smoking, 65
Tourette syndrome, 43
Toxins, and substance-induced psychotic disorders, 112, **114**
Transdermal nicotine, **62**
Transsexualism, 97–98
Tranylcypromine, 42
Traumatic stressor, definition of, 32–33
Trazodone
aggression and, **210**
dementia and, **88,** 89
sexual function and, 153
sleep disorders and, 181, **182**

Treatment. *See also* Medications; Psychotherapy
of anxiety disorders, 36–44
of cognitive disorders, 86–90
of depression, 8, 18–22
of eating disorders, 194–196
of psychotic disorders, 121–126
of sexual disorders, 155–165
of sleep disorders, **172,** 181–183
of somatoform and related disorders, 100–104
of substance use disorders, 52–53, 65–74
of suicidal ideation, 203–205
of violent behavior, 209, **210**
of weight disorders, 197
Triazolam, 181, **184**
Tricyclic antidepressants (TCAs). *See also* Antidepressant medications
anxiety disorders and, 37, 42
bulimia nervosa and, 196
consultation of psychiatrists on use of, 10
depression and, 17, 19
sexual disorders and, 157, 163
sleep disorders and, 173, 183, **184**
suicidal ideation and, 205
Trifluoperazine, **123**
Tyramine, in foods, 17, 41

Upper airway resistance syndrome, **172,** 174–175
Uvulopalatoplasty (UPP), 175

Vacuum devices, and impotence, 160
Vaginismus, 163
Valproic acid, 5
Vascular dementia, 80
Venlafaxine
dementia and, **88**
depression and, 16, 19
dosage of, **12,** 16
Ventricular tachycardia, 129
Veterans, and posttraumatic stress disorder, 33
Violence and violent behavior
domestic violence and, 209
evaluation of, 207–209
general principles, 205–206
psychiatric disorders and, 206–207
treatment of, 209, **210**
Viral encephalitis, 110–111
Visits. *See* Appointments; Follow-up visits
Visual hallucinations, 108
Vital signs, and substance abuse, **54, 56**
Vitamin E, 86
Volatile substances, and substance-induced psychotic disorder, **114**
Vulvar vestibulitis, 163

Weight disorders, 196–197
Weight gain, and antipsychotics, 129
Wernicke-Korsakoff syndrome, 58, 60, 61, 81
Wilson's disease, 110

Withdrawal, from substances of abuse
  benzodiazepines and, 70–71
  nicotine and, 65–66
  signs and symptoms of, **56–57**
  treatment of, 59

Yohimbine, 156, 159

Zolpidem
  dementia and, **88,** 89
  sleep disorders and, 178, **182,** 183